U0350466

改变，从心开始

立 品 图 书 · 自觉 · 觉他
www.tobebooks.net
出 品

# 巴赫花精与自我疗愈

## 疾病的本质和治疗方法

（英）爱德华·巴赫　著

郑建萍　王慕龄　译

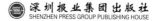

深圳报业集团出版社
SHENZHEN PRESS GROUP PUBLISHING HOUSE

责任编辑：郭良原

特约编辑：王月怡　罗　熠

装帧设计：尚上文化

**图书在版编目（CIP）数据**

巴赫花精与自我疗愈：疾病的本质和治疗方法 /
（英）巴赫著；郑建萍，王慕龄译 . -- 深圳：深圳报业
集团出版社，2015.1

ISBN 978-7-80709-649-8

Ⅰ . ①巴… 　Ⅱ . ①巴… 　②郑… 　③王… 　Ⅲ . ①香精油
－应用－精神疗法　 Ⅳ . ①R749.055

中国版本图书馆 CIP 数据核字 (2015) 第 020029 号

# 巴赫花精与自我疗愈：疾病的本质和治疗方法

Bahe Huajing Yu Ziwo Liaoyu : Jibing De Benzhi He Zhiliao Fangfa

（英）爱德华·巴赫 著

郑建萍　王慕龄　译

深圳报业集团出版社出版发行

（518009　深圳市深南大道 6008 号）

三河市华晨印务有限公司印制　新华书店经销

2015 年 5 月第 1 版　2015 年 5 月第 1 次印刷

开本：787mm×1092mm　1/16

印张：16.25　字数：130 千字

ISBN 978-7-80709-649-8　定价：45.00 元

谨以此书献给所有身心受苦的大众……

# 目　录

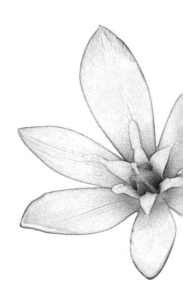

序　言　　　　　　　　　　　　　　　　/ 1

译者序　　　　　　　　　　　　　　　　/ 3

巴赫医生的生平　　　　　　　　　　　　/ 6


第一部　自我疗愈

第一章　疾病的本质　　　　　　　　　　/ 3

第二章　生命的基本原理　　　　　　　　/ 8

第三章　人类真正的痼疾　　　　　　　　/ 13

第四章　解除痛苦的良方　　　　　　　　/ 18

第五章　重要的亲子和师生关系　　　　　/ 26

第六章　听从心灵的指引　　　　　　　　/ 32

第七章　我们如何帮助自己？　　　　　　/ 40

第八章　疗愈自己是伟大的成就　　　　　/ 49

# 第二部　十二种治疗花精及其他花精

编者按　　　　　　　　　　　　　　　　　　　　　/ 60

引　言　　　　　　　　　　　　　　　　　　　　　/ 68

花精以及每种花精功能的描述　　　　　　　　　　/ 72

　　给心怀恐惧的人　　　　　　　　　　　　　　　/ 73

　　给因不确定而受折磨的人　　　　　　　　　　　/ 75

　　给不活在当下，对现况缺乏兴趣的人　　　　　　/ 77

　　给孤独、寂寞的人　　　　　　　　　　　　　　/ 81

　　给对外来影响与他人想法过于敏感的人　　　　　/ 82

　　给沮丧、绝望的人　　　　　　　　　　　　　　/ 84

　　给过度关心别人的福祉的人　　　　　　　　　　/ 88

使用指南　　　　　　　　　　　　　　　　　　　　/ 91

　　花精的使用方法　　　　　　　　　　　　　　　/ 91

　　配制方法　　　　　　　　　　　　　　　　　　/ 93

附录 1　花精的英文名、拉丁名及中文名　　　　　　/ 97

附录 2　第一部英文版 Heal Thyself　　　　　　　　/ 101

附录 3　第二部英文版 The Twelve Healers and

Other Remedies　　　　　　　　　　　　　　/ 173

# 序　言

爱德华·巴赫于 1930 年，在英国威尔士的阿伯索赫撰写了这本书的前一部分《自我疗愈》。该书的原名为《走到阳光下》。从第一章提到佛陀，到最后一段涉及灵性境界至高的圣人先贤，整本书贯穿了同一个主题——把光带给全人类。

在撰写前一部分之前的几个月，巴赫医生就已离开伦敦，全心致力于这日见雏形的花精治疗体系，当时他仅发现了配制花精的日晒法。几年后，他完成了所有的研究工作，较早版本的《自我疗愈》一书的某些观点有所变化。在第三章中，具体身体症状和情绪之间的关系被证明不完全靠得住，特别是当你决定选择或放弃使用花精的时候。他当时提到的关于"未来的医生"的观点是针对医生的，而不是他们的病人；而到 1932 年，他意识到：我们都是疗愈者。
感谢花精！

《自我疗愈》的中心思想依然与当今的咨询师及花精使用者息息相关。本书主要阐明巴赫医生关于医药、灵性、健康和疗愈的见解，其中很多主要概念对于引导他的研究而言是至关重要的。值得重视的是，在他所有的著作里，他最希望这部分内容以及《十二种治疗花精及其他花精》能留传给后人。

斯蒂芬·鲍尔

英国巴赫中心

2013 年 11 月

# 译者序

　　我们俩分别从中国湖南医科大学、台北医学大学踏上探寻人类健康之路，除了花精，我们涉足的领域还有西医、西药、中医、公共卫生学、顺势疗法、心理治疗、香薰疗法、瑜伽、禅修、心理学、人智医学、哲学、宗教。我们发现健康是先从心灵开始，而疗愈也应该是从里到外。

　　从 20 世纪 70 年代开始，医学领域对健康与疾病的阐述，从生物医学模式转变为生物、心理、社会模式，承认人的情绪、人格特质对健康有直接的影响。英国的爱德华·巴赫医生于 1933 年创立的巴赫花精治疗体系不但阐述了这些原理，还研制出一整套花精，用以调节情绪、纠正人格的不圆满，实现从内向外的疗愈。物质世界在变迁，人们喜怒哀乐的原由发生了改变，但古人的喜怒哀乐与现代人的喜怒哀乐是一样的，具有同样的本质。所以，这套疗愈体系创立八十多年，仍然完整、实用、有效，并已流传到世界各地。

由巴赫医生亲自撰写的《自我疗愈》、《十二种治疗花精及其他花精》两部分内容是该体系的核心。我们渴望能精确、准确地翻译出来，使更多的人受益。为了方便有需要的读者参考，我们还将英文原著附在了书后。如果这本书能如巴赫医生所期望的，成为每个人的枕边读物，从而达到了解自己、理解他人和疗愈自己、帮助他人的目的，那么个人、家庭以及人类社会的健康就能早日实现。

在实践花精咨询的过程中，我们不但亲身体验了花精带来的益处，也目睹了众多求助者的生活发生了积极的改变。有个叫贝力的 6 岁女孩，跟妈妈参加活动的时候总是躲在妈妈身后，问她为什么，她说害怕。这种害怕阻碍了她的参与，从而阻碍了她的学习和成长。贝力服用构酸酱后，她父母高兴地看到贝力开始变得大方、爱笑，积极参与团体活动了。有个孤独的父亲服用水堇后说："与人交往，我开朗一些了（周围有朋友也这么说），我觉得这是我服用花精后自我感觉发生的最大变化。"

　　巴赫花精治疗体系近几年才开始被介绍到中国来，并立刻受到欢迎。咨询师与广大求助者都渴望这两部分核心内容的中文版能早日出版。我们花了近两年的时间细心推敲、精心审校，使得本书中文版得以成熟。感谢北京立品图书有限公司，使得本书能与读者见面。

　　本书的翻译得到台湾从事巴赫花精临床咨询与教学多年的张伊莹女士、广州体育大学的周兰君副教授、北京大学的徐丹丹老师的细心审校与指正，以及澳大利亚阿德莱德大学的霍米·阿泽米汉博士和英国巴赫中心斯蒂芬·鲍尔先生的指点。在此特表感谢。

郑建萍

医生、家庭咨询师、国际注册巴赫花精咨询师（BFRP）

2014 年 4 月 2 日

澳大利亚昆士兰州

王慕龄

博士、国际注册巴赫花精咨询师（BFRP）

2014 年 4 月 2 日

中国北京

# 巴赫医生的生平

1886 年，巴赫医生出生于英国伯明翰的一个小村庄，从小直觉敏锐、文质纤巧、独立并热爱大自然，能感受到所有生命承受的痛苦并产生深切的同情，所以后来决定学医。先后就读于伯明翰医学院和伦敦医学院，取得了内科医师、外科医师学位，之后又在剑桥大学取得公共卫生学的学位。

成为一名医生后，巴赫医生曾在伦敦的一家私人诊所工作，在那里，他有了自己的实验室，并作为细菌学专家和病理学家开始研究疫苗。

繁重的医疗工作加上研究和教学，使巴赫医生在 1917 年罹患了恶性肿瘤。他的同事为他做完切除手术后，预言他只剩下三个月的寿命。一等到能下床，巴赫医生就回到了实验室，决定在余下的时间里尽快推进自己的研究。几个星期过去，他的身体越来越好，三个月过后，他却比以前更健康了。他相信是自己在做着自己的内心渴望做的事情救了他，从而推论出做自己真正喜欢做的事情是身心健康的必要因素。

巴赫医生的疫苗研究尽管顺利，但他对人们对医生的期望——只专注于疾病而忽视整个人——感到不满，多年的临床经验使他了解到情绪、人格特质对健康的直接影响，他认为疾病是源于深层次的生命失调，所以只针对症状进行治疗是不够的。他决心寻找一种更为整体的治疗方法，虽然还未成为顺势疗法治疗师，他还是进入伦敦皇家顺势疗法医院工作，很快就发现了自己的疫苗研究与顺势疗法原理之间的相似之处，并从细菌中研制出了七种病质药。

到那时为止，巴赫医生一直在研究细菌，虽然成绩斐然，但他希望找到不只针对症状进行治疗、更天然纯粹的治疗方法。受到顺势疗法的启发，他开始搜集植物，希望以更为温和的药物代替病质药。1928 年，巴赫医生在威尔士郊外发现了最早的两种花精植物——凤仙花和构酸酱。

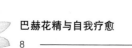

1930 年，他放弃了伦敦待遇优厚的工作，回到乡村继续花精的研究。他确信自己能从大自然中找到一种新的疗法，决心竭尽余生去寻找。

巴赫医生认为，从远古以来，一切生物都知道预防与治疗疾病的天赐手段已被安置于大自然之中，在被赋予了特别能力的花草树木里。在大自然中，他敏锐的感知力和直觉不断将他引向合适的植物。经过多年的试验，准备并检测了几千种植物，克服了种种误差，他终于一个接一个地找到了他想找的药方，研制出 38 种花精，每一种都对治一种特定的心理状态或情绪。当他用花精治疗病人时，他们内心的不快乐和身体上的痛苦都会自然而然地减轻，因为花精能调和负面情绪，引导出病人内在的自我疗愈潜能，并使这种潜能一再地发挥作用。

1930 年到 1934 年间，巴赫医生的生活遵循着四季的节律：春夏时寻找并制做新的花精，冬天则向找他的所有人提供帮助和建议。

1931 年，巴赫医生出版了阐述其医学理念的著作——《自我疗愈》。1934 年，巴赫医生和他的助手诺拉·威克斯搬到牛津郡的维农山庄（后来成为英国巴赫中心所在地）居住和工作。在那里，他经历、体验、承受了各种负面情绪在自己身上的直接影响，并在花精的帮助下一一得到调和，完成了整套巴赫花精治疗体系，于1936年9月出版了《十二种治疗花精及其他花精》，然后在1936年11月27日晚上于睡眠中过世。

巴赫花精从开始生产，就被英国药品监督机构划定为食品或饮料，人们可以以低廉的价格轻易地买到。巴赫花精应用广泛——从新生儿到老人，从慢性病、临终关怀到女性美容领域，适用于各个年龄层的人和多个领域，实现了巴赫医生想要利益众生的心愿。现在，巴赫花精已传播到世界各地，并启发出北美花精、澳洲花精等许多新的系列。

# 第一部
## 自我疗愈

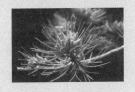

# 第一章　疾病的本质

　　本书的目的并非要否认医术的必要性，根本没有这样的想法。而是虔诚地希望本书能引导受病患折磨的人们，向内寻找患病的根源，从而帮助人们进行自我疗愈。更祈望本书能激励那些心怀人类福祉的医务工作者和宗教团体，加倍努力，寻找减轻人类病痛的良方，让人类得以早日彻底克服疾病。

　　现代医学失败的主要原因是它只处理疾病的结果，而没有从疾病的根源入手。几个世纪以来，人们因受物质主义的遮蔽而看不清疾病的本质。正因为始终没有击中病因，于是疾病得以横行肆虐。这情形就像敌军在山谷间安营扎寨，建起了坚固堡垒，从那里不断派兵四处袭击，烧杀掠夺。而受害的百姓只知修复因袭击受损的房屋，掩埋被侵略者杀戮的同伴，却不知对抗敌方基地。总体而言，这就是当今医学的情形：修复损者，掩埋死者，而从未想过疾病的真正据点所在。

当前的物质主义方法是永远不能治愈或根除疾病的，原因很简单，疾病的根源并非物质本身。我们所知的疾病是源于深层次的生命失调，即更高意识与个性不和谐的最终结果，是深远持久的压力长期作用的最后产物。即使物质手段好像看起来很成功，但如果真正的病因没有清除的话，那只是暂时地缓解病情。现代医学通过对疾病本质的错误诠释及专注于身体的物质层面，使物质主义的医学理念危害更深。首先，它干扰人们的思想，使人们找不到真正的病因，从而无法实施有效的治疗。其次，它把病因局限在身体层面，使人们看不到恢复健康的希望，还衍生出一种强大的疾病——恐惧症。事实上，这种恐惧根本是莫须有的。

**疾病的本质是人的灵魂与思想冲突的结果，除非采用精神和心理治疗手段，否则永远无法根除。**这些手段如果在正确理解下得到恰当应用，像我们随后会看到的，就可以消除基本致病因素，从而达到治疗和预防疾病的效果。

任何单纯针对身体的治疗手段都不过是表面上的修复，不是疗愈，因为病根依然存在，随时可能会以另一种形式表现出来。事实上，许多临床案例表明，表面上的恢复是有害的，因为它蒙蔽了病人，使其沉醉于表面上重获健康的满足感中。殊不知，那未被注意到的真正病因正在悄悄发展壮大。相反，有些病人自己或通过明智良医的点拨，了解到负面的精神或心理能量会促使身体产生疾病，如果这些病人直接尝试平衡这些负面能量，健康就会有所改善；一旦这些负面能量完全消除，疾病就会消失。这就是真正的疗愈：攻克据点，消除病因。

现代科学物质主义方法中的例外之一是哈内曼——顺势疗法的伟大创始人，他深刻领悟上天的无限慈爱与深藏在人类心中的神圣本性，研究病人的生活态度、生活环境及其所患的疾病，在植物领域与大自然王国里寻找药方，这些药方不仅修复身体，同时还改善病人的精神面貌。希望他所创立的学科能够被那些充满人文关怀的医师不断丰富和发展。

在基督诞生前五百年，一些古印度的医生在佛陀的影响下，将疗愈的艺术发挥到极致——他们甚至不需要外科手术，尽管当时的外科技术和今日的外科技术一样高效，有些方面甚至超过今日。正如对疗愈抱有伟人理想的希波克拉底[①]，坚信人有神圣本性的帕拉塞尔苏斯[②]，意识到疾病的根源在肉体之外的哈内曼，这些医学巨匠知悉疾病的真正本质及疗愈方法。如果世人遵行了这些伟大导师的教诲，人类近二十或二十五个世纪以来经历的无数不幸与苦痛就可以避免。但无独有偶，物质主义在西方世界的影响力强大而持久，注重实效的阻碍者叫嚣的声浪盖过了深知真理者的忠告。

简单说来，疾病看似残酷，实际上它是仁慈的，是对我们有益的。**如果疾病得到正确解读，它将引导我们找出自己的主要问题**。如果得到恰当处理——消除这些主要问题，我们就会比原来更健康、更圆满。病痛是在提醒我们人生的有些功课我们没有学好，直到我们掌握后，疾病才会彻底根除。还有一点需要知道的是，有些人明白且能看出疾病的征兆，如果这个时候施予恰当的精神与心理纠正

---

① 希波克拉底（约前460—前377），被西方尊为“医学之父”的古希腊著名医生、西方医学奠基人。

② 帕拉塞尔苏斯（1493—1541），中世纪瑞士医生、炼金术士、医药化学运动的始祖，其学说在十六、十七世纪有很大的影响。

手段，就可以防范疾病的发生或在病发早期根除疾病。但不管怎样，即使病情很严重，都不要绝望，只要还拥有生命，就意味着主宰一切的灵魂还有希望。

# 第二章　生命的基本原理

要了解疾病的本质，需要先了解一些基本原理。

**第一条原理：**人是有灵魂的，灵魂是人的真实自我，它也被称为神性、存有、造物之子，而身体是灵魂在地球上的居所，反映出最微弱的神性之光。灵魂就居于其中并围绕着我们，灵魂会依其意愿安排生命路线，只要我们允许和愿意，它将指引、保护、鼓励我们，警觉地、仁慈地指引我们向最好的方向走。灵魂，我们的"更高自我"，是全能存有的一个光点，是不可战胜且永生不灭的。

**第二条原理：**人来到这个世界的目的是通过人世间的生活来获取知识与经验，借此发展我们欠缺的美德，纠正缺点，完善人格，使我们的本性日臻圆满。灵魂知道什么样的环境和情况能最好地帮助我们达到此目的，因此，要将我们放置于最适合达到这个目标的道路之上。

**第三条原理：**我们必须意识到，在地球上的短暂旅程——我们所知的生命，不过是生命进化过程中的短暂一刻，就像学校里的一天。尽管我们只能看到和理解当下的这一天，但直觉告诉我们：人的诞生距生命的开始有无限之遥，人的死亡离生命的结束也有无限之远。人的灵魂——真实的自我，是永恒不灭的；而我们所能感知到的肉体却是暂时的，如我们旅行所驾乘的马匹，或完成一项工作所用的工具。

**第四条原理：**只要人的灵魂与他的人格特质是和谐的，就有喜悦、和平、快乐和健康。当人格偏离了灵魂设定的轨道，或是被自己的世俗欲望所驱使，或是被他人的游说所左右，便会产生内心的冲突。这个冲突就是疾病与痛苦的根源。不论我们在世间的职业为何——擦鞋匠或君王、地主或农夫、富人或穷人，只要我们是依灵魂指令行事，一切都会安好。我们可以进一步确信，无论我们被安放在何种境遇之中——尊贵的抑或卑贱的，都有此时此刻我们所需要学习的功课与体验，都是最有利于我们自身成长和发展的。

　　**第五条原理**：明白万物一体，息息相关，不可分割。造物主以爱来创生万物，我们所认知、感知到的一切事物，无论是一个星球或一粒石子，无论是夜空的星星或晨曦中的露珠，无论是人类还是其他低级生命，都以其无尽的形式体现着造物主之爱。下面的比喻可让我们对这个概念略见一斑：想象我们的造物主是一颗散发仁慈与爱的骄阳，向四周放射出无数的光芒，人类自身以及我们感知到的一切都是这些光线末端的粒子，被释放出来以获得经验和知识，但最终都要回到那神圣中心。尽管对我们而言，每一道光线都看似独立和独特，但实质上它们都始自同一光源，分离是不可能的，一旦光线与源头分离，它就不复存在了。因此，我们不难理解光线的分离与独立是不可能的，尽管每一道光线有其独特性，但它仍然是伟大源头的一部分。所以，任何对抗我们自身或他人的行为都会影响到整体。因为，任何局部的不完美都会通过整体呈现，而每一个局部的个体最终都必然回归完美。

　　**我们会看到两大根本性的错误**：一是我们的灵魂与人格相分离，并渐行渐远；二是对他人残暴或恶意相待，这是违背整体性的，是一种罪恶。这两者都会带来内心冲突，并最终导致疾病。明白自己错在哪里（我们通常意识不到），并努力去纠正缺点与错误，这不仅会带来喜悦、平和的人生，也有益于健康。

疾病本身是有益的，是要将我们带回到人生正轨，使我们的人格与灵魂的神圣旨意和谐一致。可见，疾病是可以预防和避免的，如果我们能认识到所犯的错误，并通过修正我们的想法和观念，就不必要忍受病痛的折磨。在采用最后的手段——病痛与折磨——之前，神圣力量会给我们各种机缘来修正自我，回归正途。我们在抗争的也许不是今生的错误或在学校这一天的错误，尽管我们的头脑意识不到自己为何会承受这些看似残酷或无缘由的痛苦，但灵魂（真实自我）清楚全部的目的，并引导我们从中获得最大益处。知悉并纠正自己的缺点与错误将缩短病程，帮助我们恢复健康。知悉灵魂的目的并默默遵从，就可以从尘世的苦难与悲痛中解脱出来，在喜悦与快乐中自由地成长。

人会犯的两大错误：其一，不遵从灵魂的旨意；其二，违背整体性。就前者而言，不要轻易评判他人，因为对某个人来说是对的，而对另一个人来说也许是错的。比如商人的工作是建立庞大贸易，不仅自己受益，也要惠及其员工。他需要获取高效管理与控制方面的知识，并发展与此相关的美德，这与为照顾病人做自我牺牲的护士所需要的特质与美德势必会有所不同。如果两者都遵行其灵魂的旨意，就能正确习得个人发展所需的品质。对人类而言，最重要的是：遵从通过良知、本能、直觉倾听到的灵魂（更高自我）的指令。

因此，从疾病的重要原理和本质来看，疾病既能预防，又可治愈。灵性治疗师和医生的工作除了给予药物外，还要传授知识，帮助人们认识到疾病是由于自身的缺点产生的，以及用何种方法能纠正或消除这些缺点，从而引领人们回到健康与喜悦之路。

# 第三章　人类真正的痼疾

我们所知的疾病已经是内在失衡的末期表现，如果要确保治疗完全成功，只处理末期症状显然无效，除非根本病因也同时被清除。人类可能犯的错误之一就是违背整体性，这源于自私的爱，因此，我们也可以说只有一种基本的痛苦——不适或疾病。违背整体性的行为可分为几种类型，而作为这些行为的结果而产生的疾病，也据此分为几大类。疾病的真正本质，将指引和协助我们去发现哪些行为违背了爱与整体性的神圣法则。

如果我们本性中充满对万物的爱，那么我们将不会造成任何伤害，因为爱会止息伤人的行为和念头。但我们还没有达至完美境界，如果达到，我们也就没有必要活在今世了。所有的人都在向完美境界探寻和发展，身心磨难实际上是在引领我们走向这个理想状态。如果能正确解读自己遭受的磨难，不仅可以加快前进的步伐，还可以使自己免除疾患与烦恼。一旦我们汲取人生的教训，消除自身的缺点，纠正工作就没有继续的必要了。必须要牢记的是：疾病本身是有益的，它在我们走错人生方向的时候警醒我们，帮助我们加速向完美境界迈进。

**人类真正的痼疾是人格不圆满，**如傲慢、残酷、仇恨、自私、自利、无知、摇摆不定、贪婪。仔细推敲，它们都与整体性的方向背道而驰，（用现代话来说）这些人格不圆满才是真正的疾病。当我们成长到一定阶段，意识到这些不圆满的性格仍继续发展并顽固不化，沉积体内，给身体带来破坏性的影响，这就是我们所知的疾病。

首先，傲慢源于缺乏认知，不知道个体渺小，完全依赖于灵魂。人能获得的所有成功并非自身的成就，而是来自神内在的赐福；其次，是缺乏比例感，看不到个体只是造物计划中微小的一部分。傲慢总是拒绝以谦卑、屈从的态度服从造物主的意愿，而做出违背造物主意愿的行为。

残酷是对整体性的否定，认识不到伤害彼此的行为就是伤害全体，也就是对抗整体性的行为。没有人会伤害身边的亲朋好友，根据整体性的法则，我们必须成长到这样的高度：意识到每个人都是整体的一部分，把所有的人都当成亲朋好友，甚至对迫害我们的人也只升起爱与同情。

仇恨与爱相对立，与造物法则相悖。它违背整个神性构架，否认造物主的存在；这只会产生出违背整体性的行为和思想，以及与爱相对立的事情。

自私自利也是对整体性的否认，没有对自己的同胞尽到先人后己的责任，反而置自己的利益于他人之上，不去关心和保护身边的人。

无知是不懂得学习，机会来时拒绝正视真理，从而在黑暗昏昧中做出许多错事。因为当真理与知识的光芒环绕我们的时候，这些错误是不可能发生的。

当我们拒绝倾听心灵的声音，就会导致摇摆不定、优柔寡断、意志薄弱，这些弱点会使我们背叛他人。如果我们明白战无不胜的神圣本性实际上就是自己，这种情形就不可能发生。

贪婪会导致对权力的欲望。这是对每个灵魂独立性与自主性的否定。每个人来到这个世上，是根据其灵魂的指引在人生道路上自由发展，增强自主性，不受阻挠地自由工作。而贪婪的人没有认知到这点，反而想去命令、塑造、指挥他人，夺取造物主的权力。

这些就是真正疾病的例证，是所有苦难与痛苦的根源和基础。如果这些违背灵魂声音的人格特质持续存在，就会产生内在冲突，这些冲突必然会通过身体反映出来，形成某种特定的疾病。

**我们现在可以知道，我们可能罹患的任何一种疾病都将引导我们发现病痛后面的人格不圆满。**比如，傲慢是思维上的自负与固执，会导致躯体僵硬、不灵活等疾病。疼痛是残忍的结果，病人通过体验自己肉体或精神上的痛苦，学会不将残忍强加于别人之上。仇恨表现的病症是孤独寂寞、脾气暴躁失控、精神混乱和歇斯底里。过度关注自我会导致诸如神经官能症、神经衰弱以及类似的病症，从而夺走生命中的诸多喜悦。无知与缺乏智慧会给日常生活带来许多困难，此外，若机会来时，仍继续拒绝正视真理，近视以及视听障碍就是其自然的结果。人内心的不稳定也会带来身体的不稳定，出现身体运动与协调的失衡。贪婪与支配他人的结果是使患病者成为自己躯体的奴隶，身体的疾患可束缚其欲望与野心。

　　**进一步来看，身体某个部位产生病痛并非偶然，而是依循因果法则，同时也在指引我们去提升。** 例如，心脏是生命的源泉，爱也是从这里泉涌而出，当人性中的爱没有成长或被误用的时候，心脏就会出问题；手的病痛表示行为不当或错误；大脑是控制中枢，如果脑部出问题，就意味着其人格缺乏控制。我们应该遵循这些因果法则。我们都承认，强烈情绪波动和惊闻噩耗之后会感到诸多身体不适。试想，如果琐事能影响身体健康，那么灵魂与身体的长期不和与冲突对我们的影响将有多严重、多深远？结果会导致今日多少悲惨的呼声和疾病，我们还会对此感到诧异吗？

　　但不必因此而沮丧。**通过找出我们内在的不圆满与错误，真心诚意培养美德，从而摧毁、根除那些缺点，就能预防与治疗疾病。** 这种方法不是去对抗缺点与错误，而是培养正向的美德，使之如滚滚洪流冲刷掉我们人性中的缺点。

# 第四章　解除痛苦的良方

我们看到，无论是疾病的类型还是影响到的身体部位，疾病的发生都并非偶然。就像所有的能量定律，疾病同样遵循因果法则。某些疾病是由直接的物理原因所致，如中毒、事故、外伤以及不节制行为。但总的说来，如前文所述案例，疾病是源于我们本性中的一些基本错误认知。因此，一套完整的治疗不仅包括物理手段——选择已知最好的疗愈方法，还包括要尽最大的努力去除自身的缺点。因为，最终完整的疗愈是从内而发，源于灵魂深处，当这些障碍被清除后，造物主的仁慈大爱就会透过我们的人格散发和谐之光。

**所有的疾病都有一个根源，即自私。**因此，也有一个特定的方法来解除所有的苦痛：将自私自利转变成奉献、服务他人。如果我们能充分培养关爱他人的美德，将"小我"融入到"大我"之中，享受自我成长、助人为乐的愉快过程，我们个人的悲伤与痛苦就会即刻烟消云散。人生的终极目标是：在为人类服务的过程中放下个人利益。无论造物主把我们放在什么位置——从事贸易或专业工作，富贵或贫穷，君王或乞丐，每个人都能在做好自己本职工作的同时，向周围的人传播"四海皆兄弟"的神圣大爱，成为他人名副其实的良师益友。

但绝大多数人在达到完美状态之前还有一些路要走，如果足够努力，达到目的地的速度也是惊人的。以世上伟大先知为榜样，并满怀对他们教诲的绝对信心，而非跟随自己不完善的人格特质，一切就都是可能的，这样我们就能与自己的灵魂、内在神性合一。每个人或多或少都有妨碍自己进步的缺点，我们必须从自身找出这些缺点，努力发展出本性中对世界的大爱，通过培养相应的正向美德消除这些缺点。起初会有困难，但也只是在最初，当我们与内在神圣本性连接时，这神圣本性就会辅助我们以惊人的速度发展出正确的思维和行为模式，只要我们坚持不懈，就一定会成功。

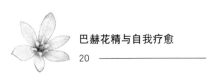

在发展内在神性大爱的同时，我们应越来越深地体悟到：每个人无论多么卑贱，都是造物主的孩子，终有一天，某个时刻，他终将达至完美，就像每个人所期盼的那样。尽管有些人或生物看起来很卑微，但我们必须要牢记，他们内在也有神性的火花，成长的过程尽管缓慢，神圣荣光终会在他们身上闪耀。

而且，是非对错的评判完全是相对的。对土著人来说在自然演进过程中是正确的东西，对于更开化的文明社会来说也许是错的；对我们来说是美德，但对圣徒来说则可能是极为不当或错误的。所谓错误或邪恶，只是善未在其位，所以万事都是相对的。请记住，我们理想的标准也是相对的，对动物来说我们俨然像神一样，然而与那些尽其一生给人类做榜样的杰出圣贤者相比，我们又远在圣者的标准之下。因此，我们必须对最卑微的人怀有悲悯之心，或许我们觉得自己比这些人优秀很多，但实际上我们也是微不足道的，与圣人之境相距甚远，他们的光辉世代闪耀。

如果被傲慢所困，我们需要明白，人是非常渺小的，除非借助于灵魂之光，否则，我们是无法做到除恶扬善的。我们更需要了解造物主的全能与强大，从滴水世界到宇宙的层级体系都是他完美创造的体现。在他面前，我们是多么地卑微渺小，完全仰赖于他。我们要懂得去崇敬、尊重人类的智者先贤，我们更应该在整个宇宙的伟大建筑师面前，以极大的谦卑承认自己的脆弱与渺小。

如果被残酷或仇恨所牵绊，请牢记：爱是创生的基石。每个生命都有好的特质，最好的人也会有缺点。努力发现他人的善，即便对那些曾经冒犯我们的人，也应培养基本的怜悯之心，祝福他们能走上更好的道路并升起助人向善的渴望。最终战胜一切的是爱与仁慈，当我们充分培养出这两个特质之后，凡事都击不倒我们，因为我们全身洋溢着的是同理心，而不是对抗，因果法则再次证明对抗的结果是伤害。我们生命的目标就是遵循自己心灵的指引，不受外界干扰。要想达到此境界，我们必须温和地走自己的路，同时不用任何残酷或仇恨的手段去伤害或干预他人。我们必须尽最大的努力去爱他人，也许从爱一个人甚至从爱一个小动物开始，让爱发展延伸至更广的层面，直到所有的负面特质自动消失为止。爱衍生爱，恨增长恨。

**治疗自私的有效方法是将对自我的关心与专注转向他人，在专注于为他人谋福利的过程中忘却自我。**正如一位

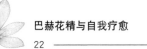

伟大先贤所说："解除我们痛苦的良方，是在同胞受难的时候去安慰、帮助他们。"世间没有比这更有效的方法来治疗自私自利以及随之而来的身心失调。

根除摇摆不定的良方是培养坚定的意志，下定决心，坚定执行，杜绝犹豫不决、摇摆不定。即使最初会犯一些错误，但行动总比为了等待"正确"决定而错失良机好得多。决断力会不断成长，害怕陷入生活的恐惧会消失，从行动中获得的经验将引导我们作出更好的抉择。

要消除无知，就不要害怕去亲身体验。时刻保持头脑清醒，睁开眼、打开耳，尽可能地吸收知识。同时思想要灵活，以免先入为主的想法以及固有的信念妨碍我们汲取更新、更广的知识。我们应随时准备好打开心扉，放下根深蒂固的成见，在体验人生的过程中让真理自然展现。

跟傲慢一样，贪婪也是阻碍我们进步的一大障碍，这两者都必须要毫不留情地铲除。贪婪的恶果非常严重，它使我们干预他人灵魂的成长。我们必须要认识到，每个人来到世上的目的是听从其灵魂的指引，使自身日臻圆满。除了其灵魂之外，谁都不能干预其发展，只能给予鼓励和支持。我们应尽力帮助他们增长知识，获得世俗的经验以提升生命。正如我们希望在人生的道路上能获得别人的帮助，以度过艰难的时期一样，我们也应准备好随时伸出援手，将我们的经验传授给需要的人。父母对子女、老师对学生、同侪之间也应持这种态度，在对方需要的时候给予关怀、爱和保护。重点是让每个生命依其灵魂的指引，自由地发展他的人格特质，绝不在任何时刻阻碍其发展。

大多数人在幼年期比成年期更容易接受心灵的指引，更清楚该做什么，该朝什么方向努力以及该发展什么样的人格特质。成年后迷失的原因在于，当今的物质主义潮流、时代背景以及与我们关系紧密的人使我们倾听不到内心的声音，偏离心灵指引的道路，缺乏理想抱负，被困在平庸之中，这在当代文明世界中屡见不鲜。父母、老师、伙伴要尽力鼓励身边的人注重心灵的成长，因为这些人拥有更多的特权与机会对身边的人施加影响。予人自由，就像自己渴望拥有自由一样。

同理，我们要努力找出自身的不圆满，通过培养相应的正面特质来去除这些不圆满，化解灵魂与人格的冲突，这些冲突正是疾病的根源。如果有坚定的信心，培养正面的人格特质就可以减轻病痛，带来健康与喜悦；如果自身的信心不够，通过配合医生的治疗也可以带来同样的效果。

我们必须遵从自己内心的指引，真诚学习，发展正面的人格特质，不惧怕他人也不允许他人干扰或阻挠我们提升生命，实现自己生命的目的，并向同胞伸出援助之手。牢牢记住：我们越接近圆满，对身边的人就越是福佑。在帮助他人时要随时警醒，无论对象是谁，助人的心愿需发自内心，而不是在强势者建议或说服下生出的虚假责任感。社会公约会造就这样一种悲剧：无数儿女出于责任感守候在久病不愈的父母身边，而父母的唯一疾患就是贪求儿女的关注，从而使得多少青春被葬送，多少良机被错失，多少身心痛苦与折磨因此而产生。试想，多少热血青年的天性被捆绑，没有勇气从强悍者手中赢回自由，从而丧失了为人类做出伟大贡献的机会。孩子在生命早期知道并渴望遵从自己的天命，但由于困境、他人劝阻以及目标感薄弱而滑落到生命的支流中，结果既不快乐也无法实现个人的提升。只有我们的内在良知能告诉我们，我们今生的天职是什么，该为谁服务以及怎样服务。但无论是什么，我们都应竭尽全力遵从内心的指引。

　　最后，让我们不惧怕投入到生活中。我们今世的目的是获得人生经验与知识，除非面对现实，努力探求，否则我们将一无所获。体验无处不在，无论是宁静的乡村还是嘈杂喧闹的都市，我们都可以获得人生的经验，体会和了解自然与人性的真谛。

# 第五章 重要的亲子和师生关系

　　缺乏自主性（即个人人格的发展受到干扰，无法按灵魂的指令、内心的声音行事）是身心疾患的一大主因，这种情况通常始于生命早期。让我们审视一下父母与孩子、教师与学生之间的真正关系。从根本而言，为人父母是一项特权（事实上应被视为一项神圣的特权），主要在于帮助另一个灵魂接触世界，完善自我。正确理解的话，对人类而言，没有比成为父母更好的机会，去作为一个新生命的指引者，并在生命的最初几年关心照顾他。父母应尽自己最大的能力给这个新生命以精神、心灵及身体发展的引导。永远不要忘记，这个幼小生命是一个独立的灵魂，是根据其灵魂的指引来这个世上获取经验和知识的，应给他尽可能的自由，不妨碍其发展。

父母职责是一项神圣的服务工作，应视为比其他事情更为重要的工作。它是一种牺牲，永远记住，不要期待孩子有任何回报，一切都只为给予，只有给予，给予温柔的爱、保护和指引，直到这个灵魂人格独立。应尽早教他什么是独立、自主、自由，鼓励他尽可能独立思考与行动。随着孩子自我管理能力的逐渐发展，父母的控制应一点一点地放松。之后，不要以父母职责为由，约束或妨碍孩子倾听其灵魂的指引，这种观念是错误的。

为人父母是生命赋予我们的一项职责，从上一代传给下一代，实质上是在短暂的时间内给予新生命指引和保护，之后要让孩子不受干扰地自由成长。父母需要谨记，我们暂时对其行使监护权的这个孩子，其灵魂也许比我们更成熟、更伟大，其灵性可能远远高于我们，因而对孩子的控制与保护应以他的特质发展需要为限度。

为人父母是神圣的职责，其性质是短暂的，代代相传。除了服务与不求孩子回报外，别无其他；而孩子也应按自己意愿得到自由发展，以使自己尽可能地胜任同样的职责，因为数年后，他们也将为人父母。因而孩子不应受到限制与阻碍，不应有回报的义务，而是清晰地明白为人父母的

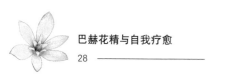

特权被先行赋予其父母，日后自己也要承担为人父母的职责。

父母尤其要避免用上天赋予他们帮助新生灵魂成长的天然职责和神圣特权，来控制孩子或索取回报。任何控制的欲望或以个人目的塑造孩子的愿望，都是贪婪的一种可怕表现，绝不支持。因为如果年轻父母早早种下这样的种子，就会使其日后变成名副其实的"吸血鬼"。即使是一丝操纵与控制的欲望，也要及早觉知。我们必须拒绝做贪婪的奴隶，贪婪促使我们想要占有他人。我们应该鼓励自己培养给予的艺术并发展这个特质，通过一次次的牺牲与奉献，将贪婪的负面特质去除。

教师应永远牢记，其职责是引路人，为学生创造机会学习与世界和生活相关的知识，使孩子们以自己的方式吸收知识。在自由的环境里，学生会本能地去选择令其生活成功的知识与技能。因而，应给学生最温和的关心与引导，帮助他获得所需的知识。

作为儿女，我们应记住，父母的责任是创造力的象征，是一项神圣的任务，不能以此限制孩子发展，也不应以义务为由，阻碍孩子追随内心的指引去生活和工作。当今的文明社会使数不胜数的人因为缺乏对这一事实的认知而默默受苦，天性被扭曲，性格变得霸道专横。

基于错误的动机和对亲子关系的错误认知，许多父母把家变成了囚闭家人的"监狱"。这些"监狱"限制自由，禁锢生命，阻碍自然成长，所有生活在里面的人都不快乐，忍受精神、心理及生理失调的折磨。事实上，当今的大部分疾病都源于此。

多数人意识不到，每个人来到今世有其特殊的目的，即获得经验与知识，在灵魂设定的目标下完善自我。无论我们彼此的关系是什么，无论是夫妻还是亲子，无论是兄弟姐妹还是师徒关系，如果我们以个人动机去阻碍他人成长进步，我们就是在违背天理，对抗自己的手足同胞。我们唯一的责任就是遵从自己良知的指引，同时绝不允许他人控制和支配我们。

让所有的人都谨记，灵魂已设定了人生之路，如果不依此前行，即使是无意识的偏离，灵魂与心灵也必会产生冲突，这一冲突会以生理失调、身体疾患的方式反映出来。

实际上，有些人的使命就是为他人奉献自己的人生，但在实施前他一定要十分确定这个呼唤是来自于内心深处，既不是被强势者所游说，也不是被所谓的责任的错误理念所误导。还要记住，我们来到此世是为了获取胜利，是来获得力量战胜想控制我们的人，从而达到这样一种境界：随着生命之河的流淌，平静而祥和地做自己该做的事情，不受任何人的干扰与影响，这种平和的引导永远是来自我们内在的灵魂的声音。

对于很多人来说，最大的战争是在自己的家里，在他们赢得今世的胜利与自由之前，首先要把自己从身边亲人的负面控制与支配下解放出来。

不论成年人还是孩子，每个人生命中都包含这样的功课——摆脱他人的控制。首先，那所谓的压迫者应被视为比赛中的对手、人生竞技场中的对垒者，如果没有丝毫痛苦，没有这个对手，我们就没有机会培养与发展自己的勇气与独立性；其次，人生真正的胜利是通过爱与温柔来获得的，这种竞赛不是用武力，而是不断培养良好天性——同情心、仁慈。如果可能的话，培养对你的对手的好感，甚至爱你的对手，他也许就会因你而改变，发展自己的美好特质，温和而平静地听从良知的召唤，不再给你丝毫的阻碍。

专制的人需要更多的帮助和指引，使他们能认识到整体性这一伟大普世的真理，理解人类一家，情同手足的喜悦。错失这些就是错失人生真正的幸福，我们要在自己能力范围之内尽力帮助这些人。需要明白一点，是我们的弱点使得他们有机会施加影响，不过这对他们没有丝毫益处。温和地拒绝他们的控制，并努力让他们体会给予的快乐，就能帮助他们完善自我。

要获得自由，赢得独立自主，需要极大的勇气和信念。即使是在最黑暗的时刻、在成功看起来似乎是不可能时，也永远不要忘记上苍之子无所畏惧。我们的灵魂只派给我们能力所及的任务，只要我们对自己的内在神圣本性有勇气和信心，胜利终将属于不懈努力者。

# 第六章　听从心灵的指引

亲爱的同胞们，现在我们知道爱和整体性是造物主创生的基础，我们也是这神圣大爱的孩子，征服过失与痛苦的永恒方法是爱与温柔。当我们明白了这一切，在这美丽的画面里，哪容得下活体解剖和动物腺体器官移植呢？为什么我们仍然那么原始和异类，以为通过牺牲动物的生命，就能逃脱自己的愚昧和错误呢？

大约 2500 年前，神圣的佛陀就已告知世人，杀生是错误的。人类虐待折磨动物，亏欠它们太多。这些不人道的行为非但未给人类带来任何益处，反而只会给人类和动物世界带来伤害与破坏。西方人脱离人类古老文明——古印度的那些美好理想越来越远。那时人们对地球所有生物的爱是如此深厚，他们接受训练并能够医治所有动物包括鸟类的疾患和伤痛。更胜于此，各种生物都有大型保护区，人们对伤害低等生命的人极度厌恶，以至于医生拒绝给狩猎者看病，直到狩猎者发誓彻底放弃狩猎行为。

不过不要指责做活体解剖的医生，他们大多都本着人道主义的原则努力工作，以期找到缓解人类病痛的良方。他们的动机良好，但智慧不足，对所有生命存在的因由所知甚少。仅有良好的动机是不够的，良好的动机必须要与智慧和知识相结合。

至于与动物腺体移植相关的骇人巫术，我们都不忍去谈。恳请全人类远远避开它，因为它比任何瘟疫都恶毒千万倍，这是违反上苍、人类和动物的罪恶行径！

即使发生一两个例外，也没必要追究现代医学的失败，摧毁它是没用的，除非我们重建一个更好的体系。事实上，在医药界，新兴大厦的基石已铺垫好，让我们专心去给这个疗愈殿堂添砖加瓦吧。指责批评当今的专业医生毫无意义，错的是体系，而不是人。陷入其中的医生们受经济利益的驱使，没有时间给病人实施安静、平和的治疗或对案例作必要的反思和斟酌，但这些施治手段应是奉献自己一生给病患者的医生们必须遵从的职业传统。帕拉塞尔苏斯曾说过，智慧的医生一天只看五个病人，而不是十五个病人。对当今普通医生来说，这是一个无法实现的理想。

一缕更好的疗愈艺术的新曙光已降临人间。一百多年前，哈内曼创立的顺势疗法如同一道晨光划破了漫长黑夜，它会在未来的医学领域里发挥重要作用。而且，目前人们已经注意到改善生活环境，提供更纯净、清洁的食物，都有助于预防疾病。还有一些运动正在兴起，旨在引导人们关注身心疾患的关联，以及通过完善思想来促成疗愈。这一切都指向了健康的光明大道，在此光芒的照耀下，疾病笼罩下的黑暗终将被驱散。

要记住疾病是我们共同的敌人，任何人若攻克了一部分，就不仅是帮助了他自己，也帮助了全人类。在彻底打倒病魔之前，必然要耗费一定的能量。让我们一起为这个目标努力奋斗，那些更健康、更强壮的人不但要做好自己分内的事情，还要在生活中协助比他弱小的同胞。

显然，预防疾病扩散、增强的首要方法是停止那些使病魔更猖狂的行为；其次是去除人格中的不圆满，正是这些不圆满使疾病能进一步入侵我们，成功做到这些就是胜利。只有先让自己自由，才能自由地去帮助别人。刚开始似乎很困难，但真正做起来并没有那么难。我们只要尽力而为，只要听从自己心灵的指引，这一切就都是可能的。生命不会要求我们做出超乎想象的牺牲，它要我们内心充满喜悦地走在人生旅程上，并造福他人。当我们离开人世时，如果世界因为我们的存在而有些许进步，那我们就不虚此行。

如果教义得到正确解读，所有宗教教义都是在向我们召唤"放弃一切，跟随我"。其真义是完全放下自我，听从心灵的指引，但这并非是某些人想象的放弃家庭和舒适、爱和享受，这种想法与真理相距甚远。一位王国的王子，享有皇室的荣耀，对他的子民、国家甚至整个世界来说，或许他是天赐之福。如果他认为进入寺院出家修行是自己的责任，那将是多么大的损失啊！生命之树的每个分支，无论是低处还是高处，都有它的位置和作用。命运的神圣指引会把我们放在最适合我们的位置，而我们要做的就是快乐圆满地完成这个位置所赋予的使命。圣人可出自工厂车间装配线上、轮船锅炉房里以及宗教团体的神职人员中。没有一个人会被要求去做超出其能力所及的事情，只要我们尽自己最大的能力培养正面的人格特质，遵从灵魂的指引，健康与快乐就将属于每个人。

在过去两千年的大部分时间里，西方文明专注于物质主义，而忽略了人性中的精神层面和人存在的本质意义。在人们的脑海里，世俗的财富、野心、欲望、享乐重于泰山，而生命的真实本质却轻如鸿毛。人存在的意义已经被一心渴求荣华富贵的焦虑所掩盖。由于没有认识到，在物质层面之上生命还有更重要的事情要做，因此无法享受到真正的慰藉、鼓励和提升，使得生活在某些阶段变得困难重重。

在过去的几个世纪里，宗教对很多人来说不过是一种传说，与其生活毫无关联，更不是自己存在的本质。有关我们内在的真实自我，以及关于前世和来世的知识，不但没有成为现世行动的指南和激励，反而对我们毫无意义。我们避开了这些生活的重要内容，把精神的概念从脑海中驱逐掉，依赖于尘世的欢娱作为痛苦磨难的补偿，企图让生活尽可能舒适。社会地位、头衔、金钱以及世俗的占有成为数世纪以来人们追求的目标，而这些都是暂时的，且只能通过处心积虑、专注于物质才能获得和占有。过去的几代人享受到的真正内在平和与喜悦程度远远低于人类应享有的水准。

当我们有了精神上的提升，灵魂和思想上的真正和谐就与我们同在，这种和谐不是通过财富的累积来获得，不论财富有多雄厚。但时代在变迁，很多迹象已显示，当代文明开始从纯物质主义转向渴望探求宇宙的真理与实相。当今，人们探求超物质真理的兴趣普遍日增，越来越多的人渴望了解是否有前世和来世，寻找用信仰和精神手段战胜疾病的方法，探寻古代教义与东方智慧。所有这些都表明，当今人类已经略微瞥见了万事万物的真相。那么，当我们看到疗愈这个领域存在的问题时，就能理解疗愈这门学科也要跟上时代的步伐，其方法要从粗浅的物质主义转变为以科学为基础的方法，而这门科学是建立在真理之上，且遵循同一个统领我们内在本性的神圣法则。

疗愈将从针对身体的物质治疗，转变为精神和心理层面的治疗。这种治疗是通过灵魂和思想的和谐，根除疾病的根本原因，必要时还将辅以物理的方法，以完成整个身体疗愈。

除非医务工作者认识到这些事实，并随人们的精神持续成长不断提升自己，否则疗愈这门艺术将由宗教的神职人员或天生的疗愈者掌握，这些天生的疗愈大师存在于每个时代，他们默默无闻，以使自己免于受到世俗偏见和传统医学的束缚，只听从其内在的指引。因此，**未来的医生将有两大职责**：首先是协助病人认识自己，指出他所犯下的根本错误，以及他品性中需要修正的部分，并引导其培养相应的美德。这种医生自己本身应是遵循自然与人类法则，了解人性的好学生，如此他才能分辨出造成患者灵魂与人格冲突的因素是什么。他必须能够劝告患者如何达至内在和谐，哪些行为违背了整体和谐并需要终止，以及发展必要的美德以去除这些缺点。每一个案例都需要仔细研究。能胜任这项工作的人，是那些倾注毕生精力于人类知识的人，他们内心充满着助人的热情，如此才能成功地承担这份荣耀和神圣的使命，为人类服务，打开患者的智慧之眼，引导他思考存在的目的，唤起他的希望、欣慰与信心，从而战胜疾病。

医生的第二个职责是给病人采用合适的疗愈方法，这种方法能帮助身体获得活力，协助心灵获得平静，拓宽其人生观，并向品格圆满努力奋进，从而达至身心灵的安详与和谐。这些疗法就在大自然里，是神圣造物主无限慈悲的赐予，以疗愈和安抚人类。一部分我们已经发现，更多的仍被当今世界各地的医生们探寻着，尤其是在我们的文明古国印度。毫无疑问，当这些研究越来越深入时，我们就能重新获得两千年前的许多知识，未来的治疗师将可以自由使用这些神奇而自然的疗法，而这些疗法本来就是上天安排，用来舒缓人类病痛的。

　　因此，要铲除疾病，有赖于人类领悟到颠扑不破的宇宙法则，并以谦卑和臣服之心顺应这些法则，使得身心和谐，获得人生真正的喜悦和快乐。而医生的工作将是协助病患获得这些真理的知识，并向他指出可以帮助他获得和谐的方法，激励他相信其神圣本性必能克服一切困难，并借助这些疗愈方法来健全其人格，疗愈其身体。

# 第七章　我们如何帮助自己？

现在，我们来谈最重要的问题，我们如何帮助自己？我们怎样保持身心和谐的状态，使得疾病很难或无法攻克我们。因为没有冲突的人格能免受疾病的侵害。

首先来看看我们的想法。我们已经长篇讨论了寻找自身不圆满的必要性，因为正是这些不圆满的人格特质，使我们与整体性相抗衡，没有顺应灵魂的指引而失去和谐。但我们可以通过发展相应的美德来纠正这些不圆满的人格特质。这些可以通过之前提到的思路实现，诚实的自我观察就能看清我们错误的本质。我们的精神导师、真正的医生以及亲朋好友应该都能协助我们看到真实的自己，但学习看清自己的最好方法是通过静思冥想，把自己带入到和平宁静的氛围中，这时候我们的灵魂就能通过我们的良知和直觉与我们对话，并依其意愿指引我们。

　　如果我们能每天抽出一点时间，找个尽可能安静的地方独处，不受任何干扰，只是静静地坐着或躺着，或者什么都不想，或者静思自己人生所为，之后就会发现这种时刻能带给我们巨大的帮助，知识与指引将如泉水般涌向我们。我们会发现，生活中的所有难题都得到了准确无误的回答，并能自信地选择正确的志业。在整个过程中，我们的心思应集中在渴望服务于人类福祉、依灵魂意愿行事上。

　　要牢记的是：当我们找出自身人格的不圆满时，解决的方法不是与之对抗，也不是用自己的意志力把它强压下去，而是坚定稳健地培养与之相对应的美德，这样我们本性中的不圆满就会被自动冲洗掉而不留痕迹。这才是真正、自然的提升方法，比单独去对抗某个缺点来得更简单有效。与恶习对抗只会增强它的力量，它会吸摄我们的注意力，让我们与之搏战，而我们能期待的最大成功不过是用压抑战胜它，但结果并不如人意，因为敌人仍跟我们共生着，会在我们虚弱的时候乘虚而入。忘掉缺点，努力培养美德，使得那些缺点无处可藏，这才是真正的胜利。

例如，如果意识到自己本性中有残酷，我们会不断地告诫自己："我将远离残酷"，不让自己偏向这个方向，但这种成功倚赖于思想的力量，一旦思想力量减弱，我们就会忘记自己美好的决心。另一方面，我们如果发展出对人真正的同情心，这个美质将使残酷无立身之地，因为深厚的同情心会使我们远避对同胞的任何残酷行为。如此，既不需要压抑，也不需要提防暗藏的敌人（被压抑的负面情绪）突然攻击，因为同情心已经从我们的本性上根除了任何伤害他人的可能性。

如前所述，身体患病的本质是通过物质层面向我们指出思想上的不和谐，这才是疾患的根本原因。所以，克服自身的人格不圆满的另一个成功因素是我们要对生活充满热情，不要把人生仅仅看成是为了责任而尽可能地耐心生活，而要在今世旅程中不断发展出真正的喜悦。

或许物质主义最大的悲剧之一是无聊感日增，内在喜悦感日减。它教导人们在世俗的享乐与快感中寻求满足，麻痹自己受伤的心，但这些除了能让我们暂时忘却苦恼外，毫无裨益。一旦我们开始在玩乐之中寻求慰藉，我们就开始了一种恶性循环。消遣享乐对我们不是坏事，但不能一味依赖。世俗的任何快感需要不断强化刺激才能维持下去，昨天是那么兴致盎然、充满刺激，明天可能就变得索然无味了。于是我们继续寻找更大的刺激，直到我们腻透了，无法再通过世俗享乐来安抚自己。这些使我们都变成了浮士德般的"享乐族"，也许在意识层面我们没有完全意识到，生命对我们来说变成了需要忍耐的责任和义务，而那种与生俱来的、理应绽放到生命最后一刻的热情与喜悦却渐行渐远。人们甚至走极端，开始通过科学手段，使用一些极端的方法来延长寿命，增加感官享乐。

无聊厌倦感会导致我们的身体罹患多种疾病，而且远比我们意识到的要多。当今这种无聊厌倦感的发生年龄越来越早，与之相关的疾病也倾向于在更年轻的阶段出现。如果我们承认有内在神圣性这一真理，清楚我们在今世的使命，从而拥有体验人生和助人为乐的喜悦，那么这种无聊感根本就不可能产生。**治疗无聊感的良药是对身边的一切都兴趣盎然，用心感受每一天，从生活中学习，认识主宰万物的真理，在学习与体验中放下自我，并在自己成长之后寻找机会帮助身边的同伴。**无论是工作还是娱乐，时时刻刻都充满学习的热情以及体验真实、探索未知的渴望。我们会发现自己可以重新从细微之中获得乐趣，曾经被认为是普通、乏味的事情，成为了我们探索与冒险的契机。大道至简，真正的喜悦来源于生活中的简单细微之处。

放弃与顺从只会让人成为生命旅程中的一个不闻不问的过客，向各种负面能量大开门户，如果我们每天意气风发，洋溢着探索生命的喜悦，这些负面能量根本没有机会入侵我们。无论身居何处，不论是城市茫茫人海中的一个工人，还是乡间山野中的一个孤独牧羊人，让我们努力将单调变成乐趣，将沉闷无聊的工作变成体验人生的喜悦良机，在日常生活中去了解人性，洞察宇宙的伟大法则。造物的法则无处不在，高山峡谷抑或身边同伴都体现着造物之功。让我们把人生变成一场新奇有趣的探险，这样，无聊厌倦感就没有了立足之地。让我们通过持久的学习，达到天人合一的和谐境界。

另一个对我们有帮助的良方是放下恐惧。事实上，在自然人类王国里没有恐惧，因为我们内在的神圣本性——真实自我——是不可战胜、永恒不灭的，如果能认识到这些，那么，作为上苍之子，我们还惧怕什么呢？在物质主义时代里，恐惧自然会因尘世躯体或外在财富而产生，因为如果这些尘世所有就是我们的全部拥有，那它们就是我们无限恐惧的因由，害怕错失攫住它们的机会，会使我们活在一种持续的恐惧中，无论是有意识的，还是无意识的。因为我们的内心很清楚，世间财富是短暂的，难得却易逝，随时都会从我们手上被夺走，我们顶多只能短暂地拥有它们。

当今时代，对疾病的恐惧已经发展成为一股强大的伤害力量，它向我们所惧之物敞开大门，使它们更容易入侵我们。这些恐惧实际上都是自私自利所致，如果我们专注于他人的幸福安康，就根本无暇去担心自己的疾患。如今，恐惧感在很大程度上促进了疾病的产生和发展，而现代科学又通过向大众散播其"医学新发现"来增强恐惧的势力范围，但事实上，这些新发现尚未被完全证实。细菌及各种微生物导致疾病的学说在人们的脑海中根深蒂固，从而心生恐惧，并更加不堪一击。科学例证或日常所见都可以证实，细菌之类的低级生命也许对身体疾患有一定影响或关联，但绝不是问题的全部真相。一个事实是，科学无法从物质层面解释，为什么暴露在同样的感染源之下，有些人会罹患疾病，有些人却安然无恙。

物质主义忽略了一个高于物质层面的因素，而这个因素在日常生活中左右着个体罹患疾病的情况，无论疾病的性质如何。恐惧本身就已经压抑了我们的思想，导致机体磁场紊乱，为疾病的入侵铺平道路，如果细菌及其他物质媒介确实是唯一致病因素的话，那人们怎么会不害怕呢？但我们发现，即使是在最严重的流行期，同处感染源下，也只有一部分人被疾病击倒。知悉真正的病因在我们的人格之中，而疗愈之方也是自我本身，我们就可以无所畏惧地前行了。

我们可以把物质媒介是唯一致病原因的恐惧抛诸脑后，因为这种焦虑只会使我们更容易罹患疾病。如果努力去营造内在的和谐，那么疾病发生的概率就不会高于我们所害怕的被雷电或陨石碎片击中的概率。

现在让我们来思考身体的本质。永远不要忘记，身体只是灵魂在尘世的居所，我们在这里作短暂的停留，是为了通过与这个世界的接触获取人生经验与知识。

不要过度认同身体就是自我，但应以尊重与关爱之心善待之，使之能健康持久，协助我们完成使命。千万不要过分关注或焦虑躯体的状况，应尽量试着去忘记其存在，将它看作灵魂与思想的载体、执行我们意志的仆人。

外部清洁与内在洁净同等重要。就外部清洁来说，西方人所用的洗澡水太烫，会使毛孔大开，让污垢进入身体，过度使用肥皂会使皮肤表面发粘。用冷水或温水淋浴，洗浴的过程中不断地将脏水换成干净的水，泡澡的过程中也要将脏水倒掉换成干净的水，这样比较接近自然的方法，也会使机体更健康。用适量的肥皂清除可见的污垢，然后用清水冲洗干净即可。

内部洁净有赖于饮食，应选择清洁、健康和尽可能新鲜的食物，主要有水果、蔬菜和坚果。要绝对避免食用肉类。首先，它会在体内产生很多毒素；其次，它会刺激食欲，使人产生异常、过度的食欲；再次，它使得我们必须对动物世界残酷无情。饮用足够的液体来净化身体，比如水、自然酿造的酒或直接取自大自然的产品，避免饮用经蒸馏处理过的人工饮料。

睡眠不应过量，因为我们大多数人在清醒时比在睡眠时更能控制自己。古话说："翻了身，就该起床了"，这是指导我们何时该起床的最佳指南。

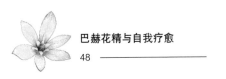

衣着应尽可能轻便，并与温度相适应，要让空气接触到身体，肌肤要尽可能多地接触阳光和新鲜空气。水浴和太阳浴可以带来健康与活力。

应多参与让人快乐高兴的事情，不要被怀疑或抑郁打击而心情郁闷，时刻记住，所有的负面情绪都不是我们的真实自我，我们的灵魂只知道喜悦和快乐。

# 第八章　疗愈自己是伟大的成就

综上所述，我们知道要战胜疾病主要有赖以下几点：第一，领悟到我们所具有的神圣本性及其所带来的力量可以克服所有的人格不圆满；第二，知晓疾病最根本的原因是我们的人格与灵魂不和谐；第三，以自身的愿望和能力去发现造成不和谐的不良人格特质；第四,通过培养相对应的美德，来修正这些不圆满。

疗愈的工作是协助我们获得必要的知识和手段，以战胜自己所患的疾病。此外，要同时服用可强化身心的良药，帮助我们更好地战胜病魔。这样我们才真正能够在疾病的最早期消灭它，拥有康复的希望。未来的医学院将不再把关注点放在疾病的最后结果和症状上，也不会过于关注实际的生理症状或给病人服用仅仅只能减轻症状的化学药物，

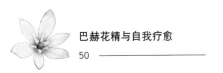
而是明白真正的病因是什么，知晓明显的身体症状仅是次要的，重在促进患者的身体、思想与心灵的和谐合一，从而缓解和治愈疾病。如果这些方法得到及早采纳，错误的思想得到纠正，就可以防止危急病痛的发生。

疗愈所采用的良方将取自大自然药房中最美丽的植物和草药，它们被上天赋予了神圣的疗愈力量，来强化人类的身心。

我们自己要做的是保持内心的和平、和谐、自主和对目标的坚定，并逐步领悟我们源自上苍，是上苍的孩子，认识到我们内在的神圣本性，长此以往，我们终将实现圆满。我们需要不断强化这一认知，直到它成为自己存在的最显著特征。我们必须坚定地实践内心和平，想象我们的心是一池平静的湖水，没有波浪和涟漪干扰，要逐渐达至这样的境界，即在任何情况下都没有任何人、事和境遇能使我们失去平静，或让我们躁怒、抑郁与疑惑。

每天留出一点时间给自己，静静地感受和平与宁静的美妙，明白担心或急躁都不能成事，而只有当我们的思想安宁、平静时，我们的行动才最有效率。让今生的行为与我们内在灵魂的愿望相一致，且让自己保持在这样和谐的状态，那么世间的混乱与动荡就干扰不了我们，这实际上就是一种伟大的成就，在平和中彻悟真理。尽管刚开始看起来不可能，但事实上，只要我们耐心坚持，每个人都能达至此境界。

上苍并没有要求我们去做圣人、殉道者或名人，而是把大多数人都放在不怎么起眼的人生位置上。但他期望我们明白人生的喜悦与探索，以愉悦之心去完成内在神圣本性赋予我们的特殊使命。

对患者来说，思想的平和、思想与灵魂的和谐是康复的最好方法。未来的医疗与护理将更专注于协助病人发展这种内在和谐。不像当今的医疗、护理行业过分倚赖医疗仪器设备，弄不清病患的病情时，更多的是去频繁测量体温、不断探视。这实际上是在打扰病人，无益于病情的康复。相反，让身心安宁与放松才是康复的重点。毫无疑问，在任何小病小恙初发时，如果我们能花几个小时让自己完全放松，让自己处于心灵、思想、身体和谐合一的状态，疾病就无法入侵我们。这种时刻我们需要给自己一种特别的宁静，这种宁静就像耶稣在风暴中登上加利利湖的船只时所命令的："风平！浪静！"

　　我们的人生观取决于人格与灵魂之间的距离，二者越接近，就越和谐与平和，更高境界的真理与喜悦之光就会越发闪耀。这种境界使我们内心平稳，不因世间的苦难和灾祸而垂头沮丧，因为此境界的基础是上天的永恒真理。真理的知识也让我们确信，无论世间的灾难有多骇人，它们都是人类演进过程中的暂时阶段。即使是疾病，也是对我们有益的，是在依照特定的法则行事，最终结果是不断敦促我们向完美迈进。具备了这些知识后，我们将不会被世间的灾难困苦所压倒或感到沮丧，所有的不确定感、恐惧、绝望都会远离我们。如果我们始终能与心灵（我们的在天之父）保持连接交流，那么这个世界就是一个喜乐之地，任何负面的东西都影响不了我们。

　　我们看不到自己的浩瀚神性，也领悟不到自己命运的强大威力，更预见不到已为我们注定的光辉未来。因为如果我们都了如指掌的话，生活就不是一场考验了，人们也不去努力了，品格也就得不到检验。在我们在未领悟到自己的神圣本性、光辉未来时，仍能充满信心与勇气地去战胜世间的困难，好好生活，这就是美德。然而，通过与内在灵魂的交融沟通，我们就能保持和谐，这一和谐使我们能战胜世间的所有对抗力量，不受负面影响，不偏不倚地实现自己的人生目标。

接着，我们必须培养并发展独立自主性，将自己从世间的各种影响中解放出来，只遵从自己心灵的指引，不被任何人或事所左右，做自己的主人，在人生的大风大浪中不偏离航道，也不允许他人替我们掌舵。我们必须拥有自己绝对、完全的自由，如此，我们的所作所为甚至所思所想就完全源于自己，使自己能自由地活着并自由地给予，而这种给予完全是发自内心的、自发自愿的。

在发展独立自主的征途上，最大的考验与困难来自于身边最亲近的人，因为在这个时代，对传统的无条件服从以及对责任的错误界定已经发展到了骇人听闻的地步。我们必须增强勇气，很多人的勇气足以应对人生中大风大浪的考验，但不足以应对身边亲密者带来的考验。在判断是非时，我们必须能够不受个人感情影响，在亲朋好友面前也能无惧无畏地行事。有多少人，在外是英雄，在家是懦夫！

那些阻碍我们实现人生目标的手段是那么微妙、难以

巴赫花精与自我疗愈

54

捉摸，比如虚情假意或错误的责任感。这些为满足一己之愿望、欲望而用来奴役、囚禁我们的方法，必须要毫不留情地抛开。如果我们不想被身边的人干扰，我们就必须只以倾听自己灵魂的声音为己任。

独立自主必须要发展到至高境界，我们必须学习独立地在人生之路上行进，不依赖任何人，只接受自己灵魂的指引和帮助，掌控自己的自由，全身心投入到这个世界，尽可能多地去获取知识与人生经验。

同时，我们也必须注意不要妨碍他人的自由，不对他人有所期望；相反，在他人需要的时候要伸出援助之手，助他人一臂之力。如此，我们生命中遇到的每个人，无论是母亲、丈夫、孩子，还是陌路人或朋友，都将成为我们人生之路上的旅伴。由于每个人的灵性成长阶段不同，有些人可能比我们强，有些人可能比我们弱，但我们都是人类大家庭的一员，是同一整体的一部分，一同经历这趟人生之旅，拥有同样的光辉未来。

我们胜利的决心要毫不动摇，登上顶峰的意志要坚定不移，不要对沿途中的偶尔失误有丝毫后悔。如果没有这些失误和跌倒，我们怎么会攀上高峰呢？这些错误都是我们宝贵的人生经验，能使我们日后少一些跌绊。不要纠结于过去的失误，它们已经过去了，结束了，而我们从中学到的知识将帮助我们免于重蹈覆辙。要坚定地向前看，往前走。不后悔，也不回头张望，甚至一个小时前的事情都应抛诸脑后，因为光辉灿烂的未来就在前方。

抛弃所有的恐惧，恐惧本来就不应存在于人的脑海中。只有当我们迷失了自己的神圣本性时，恐惧才有可能出现。恐惧对我们来说应是陌生的，因为我们是上苍的孩子，是神圣生命的火花，是不可征服、不可毁灭、不可战胜的。疾病看似残酷，它是对错误思想和错误行为的惩罚，而这些错误的思想和行为致使我们对他人残酷。因此，有必要在我们的本性中培养爱的能力和人类一家的情怀，这种大爱能将残酷彻底消灭。

爱的能力使我们领悟到整体性，感悟到每个人都出自同一个造物主。**我们所有的问题与麻烦都源于自私与分离，一旦对爱与整体性的感知成为我们本性的一部分，这些问题就会迎刃而解。**宇宙是上苍的实体表现，宇宙的诞生是上苍的重生，宇宙的终结则是上苍的演进。人亦如此，身

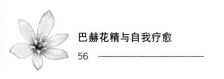
体是真实自我的外在表达、内在本性的实体表现，人是其内在本体的表达、其精神品质的物化表现。

在西方文明中，耶稣是荣耀的典范、完美的标准，他的教义指引着我们。他就像我们人格与灵魂之间的调解者，他在人间的使命就是教导我们怎样去与我们的灵性合一、与天父合一，从而依照造物主的旨意达至完美。这真理也由圣者佛陀及其他时代的先知所教导，他们向人类指明了走向完美且不可半途而废的道路。我们必须学习真理，并与造物主的无限大爱合为一体。

朋友们，让我们一起领悟自身神圣本性的荣光吧！认真坚定地准备好去努力奋斗，投身到造物主为我们设定的宏伟蓝图中，获得喜乐，传递喜乐。让自己加入到圣贤的行列，其存在的目的就是遵从神的旨意，其最大的快乐就是去服务年轻的生命。

爱德华·巴赫

内科学士，外科学士

英国皇家外科学院会员

英国皇家内科医学院执业医师、公共卫生学学士

# 第二部
# 十二种治疗花精及其他花精

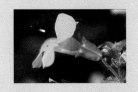

关于疗愈的研究工作已经完成并出版，我自由地给了出去，以使诸位无论病痛时还是想使自己更健康、更强壮时，都能够帮助自己。

爱德华·巴赫

50 岁生日会致词

1936 年 9 月 24 日

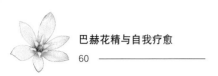

# 编者按

《十二种治疗花精及其他花精》[①]最早面世于 1930 年 2 月出版的《顺势疗法世界期刊》，当时使用的名称为《一些新花精及其新用法》。由医生转成顺势疗法治疗师的爱德华·巴赫，在期刊上发表了五种植物花精，其中的三种——凤仙花、构酸酱、铁线莲——是巴赫花精治疗体系的起始点。这些花精用顺势疗法的方法——研磨、振荡——配制而成。而用日晒法制作出我们现在所知道的花精，是在同一年稍晚的时候。

到 1932 年的时候，巴赫医生发现的花精数量已达到

---

① 1933 年初版，1934 年改版，1936 年新增版，1941 年再增版，此书为最终版。

十二种。巴赫医生就把它们收入到自己写的一本小册子里，书名为《让自己自由》。1933 年春天，他继续寻找更多花精，也有时间进一步写作与出版。其中两篇文章为《十二种极好的花精》和《十二种治疗花精》，在爱普森（Epsom）印刷。《十二种治疗花精》后来成为一本小册子，在马罗（Marlow）印刷。多年后，巴赫医生的助手诺拉·威克斯回忆起这最后的手稿在当地印成小册子的形式。他（巴赫医生）决定以两便士的价格卖给需要的人，这样人人就都能买得起，并受益于这种草药疗法。他希望这样可以平衡印刷的费用。跟往常一样，他很少有余钱，但只要有人问他要书，他就寄给他们，并总是忘记要回两便士的印刷费。

1933 年 8 月，巴赫医生写信给几年前出版了他的《自我疗愈》一书的丹尼尔公司（The CW Daniel Company），寄给他们一本《十二种治疗花精》及一份自己打印的文稿，文稿标题为"四种辅助花精"，介绍了他在那年新发现的花精。丹尼尔公司在 1933 年秋天出版了《十二种治疗花精及四种辅助花精》，并在次年，1934 年 7 月的第二版书中加进了三种花精，书名定为《十二种治疗花精及七种辅助花精》。

到 1935 年秋天，巴赫医生进一步发现了后面的十九种花精，以及配制花精的煮沸法。随着这三十八种花精的发现、配制与使用的完善，他宣布整个花精治疗体系已成熟完善了。他致信给丹尼尔公司，让他们印刷出一份两页纸的传单，介绍这些新发现的花精，并以附页形式附在原来的《十二种治疗花精及七种辅助花精》书里作为临时过渡。随后，他开始着手撰写这本书的最新、最后版本。

　　这最后的版本完全改变了原来把花精呈现给读者的程序和方式。丹尼尔公司出第一版的时候，巴赫医生曾提出这十二种治疗花精（基础花精）与七种辅助花精（这七种花精是针对长期状态，用于对十二种治疗花精的选择不明确时）有区别。现在他需要把新的十九种花精整合进原来的体系里，他推论每一种新花精也许对应先发现的一种基础花精或辅助花精。

　　这种推论模式很勉强地用了一段时间——但从未完成。也许是花精自己就落入到完美的朴素单纯模式中，与巴赫医生的感觉正中下怀；也许是某些花精自然就匹配不上。他几乎很肯定地质疑这种编排是否有任何实际应用价值："对三十八种不同人格、情绪状态的简单描述"就足以"找出病人当时表现出的某种状态或混合状态，从而给出需要的花精"①。人们最终用的是十二种治疗花精，还是那七种辅助花精，或两种都没用，或两种都用到了，真有那么重要吗？

经过大量的思考，巴赫医生完全删掉了十二种治疗花精和七种辅助花精的区别，而把三十八种花精分到七大类里。他的修改如此彻底，以致出版商担心这种改变对读者会造成影响。他们致信给巴赫医生：

我们注意到你保留了标题"十二种治疗花精"，但本书目前的格式没有标明这十二种治疗花精都是哪些。我们建议用星号（＊）标出这十二种治疗花精，并在引言里作个说明。②

巴赫医生未理会要标示出最初十二种治疗花精的要求，但在引言的结尾加了几句话来解释标题。在审校阶段，出版商自作主张地加上了星号，同时致信给巴赫医生作最后的说明：

① 巴赫医生，《十二种治疗花精及其他花精》引言，13 页。
② 丹尼尔公司致爱德华·巴赫的信，1936 年 7 月 27 日。

　　我们自作主张地在你引言补充的后面加上了这句话："最初的十二种治疗花精用星号标示出。"并在花精名称栏目和名称表部分都加了星号。[①]

　　《十二种治疗花精及其他花精》最终完成，并于1936年9月24日——巴赫医生50岁诞辰日——出版发行。根据作者的指示，出版商收回并销毁了库存的原先版本。诺拉·威克斯回忆说，一旦得出最终结论，研究结果出版发行，巴赫医生就会直接销毁他在研究过程中记录的所有手稿，这一直是他的习惯。他觉得这样就不会造成冲突，给后来者带来疑惑；他的目的是让人们明白疗愈疾病是个简单的事情，驱除人们心中对疾病的恐惧。[②]

　　1936年版本是巴赫医生有生之年的最后版本。但仅在出版发行的几周后，他就觉得该书需要改编，需要进一步捍卫这个完整体系的朴素单纯性。他致信给他的好友维克托·布伦："当《十二种治疗花精及其他花精》需要再版的时候，我们需要增加引言的内容，坚定捍卫花精的无毒性、

　　① 丹尼尔公司致爱德华·巴赫的信，1936年7月31日。
　　② 诺拉·威克斯，《爱德华·巴赫的医学发现》，第二十章。

朴素单纯性和神奇疗愈力量。"①

　　1936 年 10 月 30 日，巴赫医生将需要增加的引言口述给诺拉·威克斯，这是他有生之年最后的活动之一。一个月后，11 月 27 日，他于睡眠中过世。

　　1936 年 12 月初，诺拉·威克斯履行了其承诺，把新增补的引言寄给丹尼尔公司。1941 年版印刷时，这处改动是唯一意义重大的改动，原文全部是巴赫医生自己的原话②，该版本被认为是最后的终结版本。

　　《十二种治疗花精及其他花精》不断被印刷出版，同时也被翻译成多种主要语言——外语版并不总是成功——出版过很多版。多年来，原始的花精描述部分保持着其神圣不可侵犯性③，但原文的其他部分开放给进一步的编辑和更新。追随巴赫医生的亲自指引，巴赫中心的监护者们总是

---

　　①　给维克托·布伦的信，1936 年 10 月 26 日。
　　②　除了诺拉·威克斯对 1941 年版做的一处微小变动，见 91 页的脚注①。
　　③　唯一的例外是删除了巴赫医生对岩蔷薇描述的一句话，见正文的脚注。

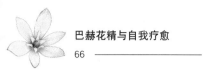
把《十二种治疗花精及其他花精》当成有生命的原文，以呈现和维护整个体系的朴素单纯性。

世界在变化，以原貌保持《十二种治疗花精及其他花精》的更新版本似乎显得没那么重要了。我们有其他的渠道呈现详尽的信息，包括剂量、对动物的作用等等：互联网、社交网络、培训课程，以及揽括了从为马匹选择花精到为自己配制的专业书籍。

当今的挑战是侧重于崇敬爱德华·巴赫的原创工作，及他对花精治疗体系未来的愿望。如果他知道 1936 年之前的版本被重新出版，且被用来重新阐述和复杂化已完成的体系，他一定会非常失望。现在，我们觉得是时候重新强调 1941 年的终极版本了，没有任何字词的删改，只是附以脚注引导读者看到原文下面的真实记录。

同时，我们与全世界范围的国际注册巴赫花精咨询师合作，以尽可能多的语种重新翻译这本重要的原著。许多目前已有的翻译版本存在严重的误译，外语终极版的准备工作已被延误了很久。

2011 年秋季是巴赫医生去世 75 周年、诞辰 125 周年的纪念日，正是奉献这份礼物的恰当时机。

茱蒂·蓝索·霍华

斯蒂芬·鲍尔

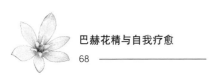
# 引　言

这套治疗体系是有史以来上天赋予人类的最完美的治疗体系①，它有治愈疾病的力量。由于其简单易行，也可以在家庭里使用。

正因为它既简单，又有全面的疗愈效果，所以如此奇妙，令人惊叹不已。

除了这里描述的简单方法之外，科学研究与专业知识不是必需的。那些保持花精的纯粹性的人将最能受益于这份天赐的礼物，摆脱科学研究与理论带来的屏障，因为大

---

① 引言的前 7 段是在 1936 年版本出版后，巴赫医生口述增加的。见"编者按"里更多的相关信息。

自然里的一切就是那么朴素简单。

这套上天揭示给我们的治疗体系告诉我们：是我们的恐惧、忧虑、焦虑以及类似的情绪，开通了疾病入侵身体的大道。因此，通过治疗我们的恐惧、忧虑与担忧等负面情绪，我们不仅不会生病，这天赐的植物还能驱走我们内心的恐惧与担忧，使我们更快乐，生活得更充实、平和。

这些植物疗愈我们的恐惧、焦虑、担忧，我们人格的弱点与缺点，这些才是我们必须要去改善与纠正的地方；当我们人格健全，内心强壮，疾病也将远离我们。

没有更多要说了的，任何头脑清明的人都会明白这些道理。希望世上有足够多头脑清明的人，不受科学潮流的羁绊，将这些天赐的礼物用于他身边的人，化解苦痛，造福人类。

所有疾病背后都隐藏着我们的恐惧、焦虑、贪婪、好恶与爱憎。让我们把它们找出来，治疗它们。在这些负面人格、情绪修复之后，折磨我们的疾病也会随之悄然离去。

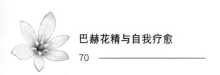

远古以来，一切生物都知道预防与治疗疾病的天赐手段已被安置于大自然之中，在被赋予了特别能力的花草树木里[①]。本书描述的各种自然花精已在无数案例中得到证实，其助人功效远远高于其同类，它们被赋予了特别的能力来疗愈所有类型的疾患与苦痛。

使用这些花精治疗病患时，不需要去关注疾病的性质。治疗的是人，人好起来之后，疾病也就消失了。健康一增长，疾病就消退了。

众所周知，同样的疾病在不同人身上会有不同的反映，需要治疗的正是这些反映，它们将引领我们去探究真正的病因。

人的心灵是人体中最精细与敏感的部分，它比肉体更早、更明确地揭示疾病的发生与进程。因而，我们选择了人的内心状态作为选择所需花精的指征。

生病的时候，人的心情和平时不一样。善于观察的人会发现，这些改变在生病之前，有时在更早之前就已经出

---

① 1936年版本的短引言是从这句话开始的。

现了。若这些改变得到及时处置，就可以预防疾病的发生。如果已经生病了一段时间，同样，患者的心情也能指引我们选择正确的花精。

不要盯着疾病不放，而是觉察个体在危急、困顿之中时，对生活的态度。

本书对三十八种不同的人格情绪状态作了简单的描述，无论是治疗自己或他人，都可以很容易地识别出当时存在的某种或几种人格情绪状态，并给出需要的花精进行治疗。

本书保留了《十二种治疗花精》这个书名①，因为很多读者已熟悉了这个名字。

花精解除人类苦痛的效果是如此确定和有益，即使在只有十二种的时候，也很有必要在当时介绍给公众，而不需要等到发现其余的二十六种，来构成完整的体系。这些先发现的十二种治疗花精会用星号标示出来。

———————————

① 这一段和下一段是在 1936 年版的审校阶段被增补进印刷文件里的，见"编者按"。

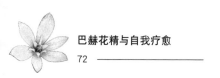

# 花精以及每种花精功能的描述

三十八种花精分述于下列七大类人格情绪状态中[①]：

1. 害怕、恐惧            73 页

2. 犹豫、不确定、茫然            75 页

3. 不活在当下，对现况缺乏兴趣            77 页

4. 孤独、寂寞            81 页

---

① 这些分类是基于巴赫医生研制的七种巴赫病质药（Bach nosodes）所确定的常见情绪特征分类。巴赫病质药是巴赫医生在1919—1928 年间研制的、从细菌中提取出来的顺势疗法药物。见诺拉·威克斯的《爱德华·巴赫的医学发现》，第五、六章。

5. 对外来影响与他人想法过于敏感　　82 页

6. 沮丧、绝望　　84 页

7. 过度牵挂别人的福祉　　88 页

## 给心怀恐惧的人

*岩蔷薇* *

属于急救花精①，可以用在看似没有希望回生的紧急情况。用于事故发生或疾病突发时，病人极度恐惧或害怕时，或事态足够严峻以致周围的人也感到惊恐万状时。如果病人神志不清，可用花精沾湿其嘴唇。此外，因情况各异还需要增加其他花精，例如，如果病人的神志不清是一种深睡眠状态，则加铁线莲；如果有（精神上或肉体上的）痛苦煎熬，则加龙芽草，等等。

---

① 这句话在本书的多数后来版本中都被删除了。巴赫医生用五种花精配成一组综合花精，称其为"急救花精"。一些读者会觉得混淆，为何这个名字也被用于描述岩蔷薇。

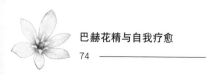

构酸酱 *

害怕具体的事物，如疾病、疼痛、意外、穷困、黑暗、
独处、不幸；害怕日常生活中的事情。这些人私下默默承受
内心的恐惧，一般不会主动向人倾诉。

樱桃李

害怕精神崩溃、失去控制；害怕失去理性，做出恐怖、
令人畏惧的事情。即使自己不愿意，也知道不对，但还是
会因为疯狂的想法和一股冲动而做出骇人的事。

白杨

模糊、无名的恐惧，解释不清楚，也说不出原因。这
类人害怕将有不祥、骇人的事情要发生，但不知道是什么。

这些模糊、讲不清的恐惧日夜萦绕，挥之不去。受此
折磨的人通常不敢将他们的烦恼告知他人。

红西洋粟

给那些很难不为他人担心、焦虑的人。

他们通常不担心自己，而是牵挂他们所喜爱的人，总是预想不幸的事情会降临在这些人身上。

## 给因不确定而受折磨的人

水厥 *

水厥典型者对自己没有足够的信心，无法为自己作决定。不断寻求他人的看法与建议，但总是被别人的意见所误导。

线球草 *

那些苦于无法在两者间作选择的人，好像左也对、右也对。

他们通常比较安静，独自承受着这种举棋不定的困境，

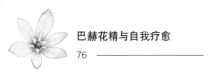

且不喜欢跟人讨论。

龙胆 *

他们很容易气馁。即使疾病有恢复或日常生活有改善，但只要有一点小小的延迟或阻碍出现，他们就会怀疑进展，而再度心灰意冷。

荆豆

非常绝望，已经放弃了所有的信念，认为再怎么做都没希望了。

他们或许会在身边人的说服下或为了迎合周围的人，而去接受某种治疗，但同时却不断地告诉周围的人：治愈的希望非常渺茫。

鹅耳枥

他们觉得自己的身心没有足够的力量，去肩负生活的责任；日常事务在他们看来似乎难以完成，然而事实上，他们通常能顺利完成每日的工作。

他们相信，要轻松地完成日常的工作，必须先强化、振奋一下身心。

### 野生燕麦

他们对生活充满抱负和野心，希望拥有丰富的人生体验，尽可能多地享受人生，让生命充实圆满。

他们的困难是不知该从事什么职业。尽管野心十足，但好像没有哪个职业让他们感到有强大的吸引力。

这既延误人生大计，又没有自我实现的满足感。

## 给不活在当下，对现况缺乏兴趣的人

### 铁线莲 *

他们喜欢做梦、心不在焉、昏昏欲睡，似乎没有完全清醒，对生活没多大兴趣。他们多是安静的类型，然而，他们对自己的现况并不真正满意、开心，更多的是活在未来，而非当下。总是幻想美好的未来，希望未来更开心，理想可以实现。如果患病的话，有些人几乎不做任何努力去恢复健康，甚至有些人期盼死去，希望死后的时光更美好，也许还可以在那里与过世的挚爱亲朋会面。

## 忍冬

他们总是活在过去，也许是沉浸在过去的某段快乐时光里，或沉浸在对过世好友的追忆中，或沉浸在自己未实现的宏伟蓝图里。他们不期待未来的日子会像过去那么美好。

## 野玫瑰

没有明显充分的理由，他们就放弃了生命中所有的挑战，逆来顺受，听天由命，不作任何努力去寻求改善、得到生命中的快乐和喜悦。他们不对生活的挑战作任何奋斗，且毫无怨言。

橄榄

已经耗尽了所有的脑力或体力，身心疲惫、倦怠，不再有一丝的力气去作任何努力。日常生活对他们来说已是沉重的枷锁，没有愉悦感。

白栗花

白栗花适用于无法阻止不想要的想法、念头、争论在脑海中萦绕，挥之不去的人。通常，在那种情况下，他们手头所做的事情单调乏味，不足以充实大脑。

那些思绪令他们担忧且挥之不去，即使暂时抛开了，很快又会溜回来。它们在人们的脑海里转来转去，带来精神上的痛苦与折磨。

这些恼人的思绪使心灵躁动不安，干扰日常的工作，使人不能享受日常生活的乐趣。

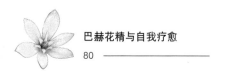

芥末

芥末适合那些容易忧郁，甚至绝望的人。当这种情绪来袭时，就好像被一片冰冷的乌云笼罩着，遮住了生命的阳光和喜悦。说不出任何原因，也解释不清楚。

在这种情形下，很难让人展现欢颜或笑脸。

白栗芽苞

白栗芽苞适用于没有充分善用自己的观察力和人生经验的人，通常他们需要比别人花更长的时间来学习生命的课程、汲取生活中的教训。

有些人经历一次就学到人生经验，而这类人需要经历几次，甚至更多次才能学到。

因此，他们经常后悔，发现自己总在不同的场合犯下相同的错误。其实犯一次错就够了，甚至可以通过观察别人，连犯一次错的机会都省掉。

# 给孤独、寂寞的人

## 水堇 *

他们不管是健康时,还是生病时都喜欢独处;非常安静,来去无声,说话很少、很轻,很独立,能力强,独立自主,几乎不受他人的意见左右。他们孤僻、冷淡,远离人群,坚持自己的原则,走自己的路。他们通常很聪明、很有天赋,他们的平和与镇静让周围的人感到非常舒服。

## 凤仙花 *

凤仙花典型者想得快,做得也快,希望所有的事情都能即时完成,绝不犹豫或拖延。如果生病了,也焦急地希望赶快康复。

对节拍慢的人很难有耐心,因为他们认为“慢”是错的,是浪费时间。他们会竭尽所能让那些“慢”的人快起来。

他们常常宁愿自己去想、自己去做,这样他们就能按自己的节拍行事了。

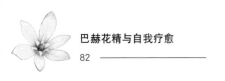

### 石楠

他们总是在寻找身边任何可能的人来与自己作伴，他们觉得必须要跟别人谈论自己的事情，且不论是谁都可以。如果他们必须独处，无论时间长短，他们都会感到非常不快乐。

## 给对外来影响与他人想法过于敏感的人

### 龙芽草 *

龙芽草典型者看似快乐且无忧无虑、幽默感十足。他们喜欢跟人和气相处，争论与争吵会令其痛苦不堪，为了不伤和气，他们宁愿放弃己见。

他们常将自己的身心不适、烦恼、忧虑掩藏在其幽默、逗趣后面，而被认为是人人愿意结识的好朋友。他们常借助过度饮酒或吸毒来刺激自己，使自己能继续用欢笑掩饰内心的苦痛。

矢车菊 *

善良、安静、温和的人，服务的愿望过于强烈。在全力以赴的过程中常让自己超负荷。

这种过于强烈的助人愿望使他们更像个奴仆，而非乐意助人者。他们的善良天性导致他们整天为他人忙碌，做了很多超出其分内的事情，以致忽略了自己人生独特的使命。

胡桃

他们对人生有明确的理想和抱负，并且会全力以赴。但倾向于偶尔会受那些热情洋溢、说服力强、很有主见的人的影响，而偏离了自己的理想、目标和所做的工作。

胡桃花精可帮助他们坚持理念，免受外界的干扰。

冬青

冬青适合那些有时被嫉恨、妒忌、报复、猜疑的念头

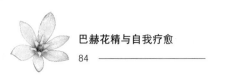

和情绪所困扰的人。

也适用于任何类型的烦恼。

他们的内心备受煎熬，而通常他们的苦恼并没有真正的原因。

## 给沮丧、绝望的人

### 落叶松

他们认为自己不如身边的人能干或有才华，预期自己会失败，觉得自己绝对不会成功。因而不敢冒险，也没有强烈的企图心作出足够的努力，去达到成功。

### 松针

他们总是在自责，即使成功了，也认为自己应该可以做得更好，对自己的努力或成果从来都不满意；他们工作辛勤努力，但总把过失全包揽到自己身上。

有时即使是别人的过错，他们也认为自己有责任。

榆树

榆树典型者忠于职守，倾听内心的召唤，希望做一些伟大的且对人类有益的事业。

当他们觉得自己承担的任务过于困难，超出常人能力时，会有阶段性抑郁、沮丧的现象。

甜西洋栗

有时人们的生命中会有这样的时刻：感到极度的痛苦，到了不能忍受的地步。

身体或心灵已经濒临崩溃的边缘，再也忍耐不了，感觉现在就要崩溃了。

眼前似乎空无一物，只有破坏和毁灭。

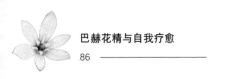

圣星百合

有些情形会给心灵带来极大的冲击，造成相当长一段时间的极度痛苦。这些情形包括惊闻重大的新闻事件、挚爱亲人的骤然离世、意外事故后的惊恐等等。

他们一时之间无法接受事实，也不愿意接受他人的安慰与关心，圣星百合花精可以抚慰他们的心灵。

柳树

柳树帮助那些面临着逆境或不幸，无法接受事实，怨天尤人的人。因为他们以人生的成功来评判生命的价值。

他们觉得自己不应该承受这么多的磨难，太不公平了，由此变得很愤怒。

他们对往日曾带给他们喜悦和快乐的事情失去了兴趣，很少参与。

橡树

如果生病了，他们会全力以赴地与病魔对抗。对日常生活中的事情也一样，尽管事情已看似无望了，他们也会一个接一个地去尝试不同的方法。

他们是斗士。如果疾病影响了他们的工作或助人之事，他们就会对自己非常不满。

他们是生命的勇士，勇敢地与困境搏斗，从不放弃希望或努力。

野生酸苹果

具有清洁净化作用的花精。

这些人觉得自己不是那么地洁净。

眼睛只盯着小病小痛：他们一旦只专注一个小毛病，对一般人觉得非常严重的疾病反而不会看在眼里。

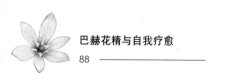

不论是不洁净感，还是小病小痛，对他们来说都是大事情，对此很焦虑，必须要尽快处理，摆脱这些困扰。

如果治疗失败，他们会很绝望。

如果病人有理由相信毒物感染了伤口，野生酸苹果花精可以净化伤口并驱除毒素。

## 给过度关心别人的福祉的人

菊苣 *

菊苣典型者脑子里想的都是别人的需要，倾向于过度关心自己的孩子和亲朋好友，总能找到事情并把它们做好，乐此不疲地把自己认为错误的事情导正。他们期望自己所关心、牵挂的人都围绕在身边。

马鞭草 *

马鞭草典型者有固定的原则和想法，一旦坚信自己是正确的，就几乎不可能改变。

他们有很强烈的、说服周围所有人认同自己的生活观的愿望。

当他们坚信某些信念并认为要教导他人时，会表现出很强的意志与勇气。

即使生病了，在别人早已放弃自己的职责的时候，他们仍在坚持不懈。

葡萄树

他们很有能力，坚信自己的才能，对成功非常有信心。

正因为如此确信，因而他们认为，说服别人去做他们正在做的事情，或做他们坚信正确的事情，是对别人有益的。即使是在病痛中，他们也会指挥那些照顾、护理他们的人。

在应对紧急突发事件时，他们能发挥极大的作用。

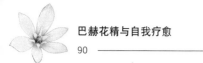

## 山毛榉

山毛榉能帮助那些希望能够看到周围人身上的善良和美丽的人。尽管很多人都有缺点和不是，山毛榉花精能增强他们的能力，去看到人性内在的良善在不断成长，且对他人不同的习性更容忍、宽容和理解，因为所有的人和事都在努力达至其最终的完美。

## 岩泉水

他们对自己的生活方式要求严格，不让自己去享受生活中的喜悦和乐趣，认为这些会妨碍他们的工作。

他们对自己立下极高的标准，希望自己成为优秀、坚强、积极的人，并不惜代价努力保持这些状态，希望自己成为众人的典范，人人向他们学习，从而成为更好的人。

# 使用指南

如果自己不能确定、选择或配制自己需要的花精，可联系巴赫中心总部<sup>①</sup> 以获得需要的治疗和花精。

## 花精的使用方法<sup>②</sup>

所有这些花精都纯净、无毒，不必担心服用过量或频

---

① 除了巴赫医生去世前口述增加的引言外，原书 34 页和 35 页是 1941 年版与 1936 年版唯一不同的地方。诺拉·威克斯将其加进来，是为了让读者知道花精（及帮助选择花精）也可以从巴赫中心获得。可参阅 1936 年版的影印版 26 页：www.bachcentre.com/centre/download/healers1936.pdf。

巴赫中心（The Bach Centre）网址为：www.bachcentre.com。

② 在后来出版的《十二种治疗花精及其他花精》里，剂量、用法被大幅度重写，以回应使用者的咨询和关注点。可比较巴赫中心 2009 年版的 23 页和 24 页：www.bachcentre.com/centre/download/healers.pdf。

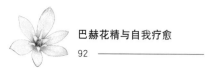

率过高。只需服用很小的剂量，就足以产生治疗效果。如果花精种类选择不当，也不会有任何伤害。

花精口服液的配制方法：从浓缩花精瓶中取两滴花精液，滴入几乎盛满水的小瓶中；如果需要保留一段时间，可加些白兰地作为防腐剂。

花精口服液可直接服用，只需几滴，和少量水、牛奶或任何饮料一起饮用都可以。

情况紧急的病人可每隔几分钟服用一次，直到情况好转；病情严重者可每半小时服用一次；病程较长的可每 2 ～ 3 小时服用一次。根据病人的感觉，可调整服用次数。

对神志不清的病人，可频繁使用花精口服液湿润其嘴唇。

身体任何部位有疼痛、僵硬、炎症或局部不适者，除口服花精外，再加上外敷花精洗液，做法是：从浓缩花精瓶中取几滴花精液，滴入一碗水中，将一块在花精洗液中浸泡过的棉布覆盖于患处。根据需要，可重复浸湿棉布覆盖患处。

在海绵沐浴擦上或泡澡的水中加几滴花精，也有效果。

## 配制方法①

花精有两种配制方法。

日晒法

取一个薄的玻璃钵，几乎盛满能找到的最纯净的水。如果可能，最好是附近的泉水。摘下盛开的花朵，迅速轻放在水面，直至花朵铺满整个水面为止。然后置放在明朗的太阳下三四个小时，或更少时间，以花朵开始凋谢作为指征。小心移除花朵，将该液体倒入玻璃瓶中至半满，然后加入同等量的白兰地防腐保存。这些液体就构成了母酊

———————

① 上世纪70年代末，诺拉·威克斯决定撤回她与维克托·布伦合著的一本关于如何制作花精的书，当中的考量是，不论用什么植物，凡是使用巴赫医师的方法来制作花精，都是属于花精整体系统的一部分。同一时期，本书的这一章节也大多被删除。1998年，巴赫中心重新出版了这本威克斯与布伦合著的书。见《巴赫花精：图解与配制》的前言。

剂①，母酊剂不能直接拿来给病人服用。必须从母酊剂瓶中
取几滴到另一个瓶中稀释后，才能用来治疗病人。因此，
母酊剂②可提供充沛的供给量。从药店买回的花精③也应以
同样的方法使用。

下列的花精用日晒法配制：

龙芽草、矢车菊、水厥、菊苣、铁线莲、龙胆、荆豆、
石楠、凤仙花、构酸酱、橡树、橄榄、岩蔷薇、岩泉水、
线球草、野生燕麦、马鞭草、葡萄树、水堇、白栗花④岩泉
水。长久以来，人们就知道某些井水和泉水有疗愈人的能力，
它们因此而远近闻名。任何因具有疗愈能力而远近闻名的
井水或泉水，如仍保持着其天然的状态，未受到人类的崇

---

① 这里，巴赫医生指的母酊剂就是"浓缩花精"，用母酊剂直接
配制花精口服液。事实上，正常的稀释过程分三个阶段：能量水与白
兰地混合做成母酊剂；从母酊剂瓶取两滴，滴入30毫升白兰地中，做
成浓缩花精；浓缩花精再稀释后就可服用。具体描述见介绍剂量的章
节。这里不清楚巴赫医生为何只把整个过程分为两个阶段，但很有可
能他觉得如果只配小剂量的花精供个人使用，则不需要中间那个环节。

② 此处的母酊剂也是浓缩花精，见上一个脚注。

③ 药店买到的花精应该是标准的浓缩花精。

④ 这里用"白栗花"，以区别同一种树上的"白栗芽苞"。白栗
芽苞是用煮沸法配制。

拜行为而污染，就可以使用。

### 煮沸法

其余的花精是用下面描述的煮沸法配制的：

将采集的植物样本放入洁净的水中煮沸半小时。过滤后倒入玻璃瓶中至半满，待凉后，加入同等量的白兰地保存。

白栗芽苞用的是白栗树上破裂成为叶子前的芽苞。

其他的是将花朵连同细枝、花茎及嫩叶一起采集。

上述的花精植物，除了葡萄树、橄榄、水厥外，其他的都自然生长在英国不列颠群岛上。尽管有些植物原生于其他地区，包括欧洲中部、南部，印度北部和西藏。

　　让我们心怀喜悦与感激，上天以无限慈爱之心，将可
疗愈我们的药草安置于大自然之中。

附录1

# 花精的英文名、拉丁名及中文名

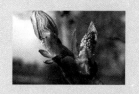

书中植物的中文名称有不同的翻译版本，下表分别列出：①

| 英文名 | 拉丁名①（植物学名称） | 现有翻译 | 本书翻译 |
|---|---|---|---|
| Agrimony | Agrimonia eupatoria | 龙芽草 | 龙芽草 |
| Aspen | Populus tremula | 白杨、火烧杨、欧洲山杨 | 白杨 |
| Beech | Fagus sylvatica | 山毛榉 | 山毛榉 |
| Centaury | Centaurium umbellatum | 矢车菊、百金花 | 矢车菊 |
| Cerato | Ceratostigma willmottiana | 水蕨、希拉图、紫金莲 | 水厥 |
| Cherry Plum | Prunus cerasifera | 樱桃李、樱花 | 樱桃李 |
| Chestnut Bud | Aesculus hippocastanum | 栗树花蕾、栗子芽、栗苞 | 白栗芽苞 |
| Chicory | Cichorium intybus | 菊苣 | 菊苣 |
| Clematis | Clematis vitalba | 铁线莲 | 铁线莲 |

① 每一种植物的拉丁名称都是按国际植物命名法规来命名的。这种法规随时代变迁而有变化，1941年用的一些名称已经过时。比如用来制作矢车菊花精的植物，过去叫 Erythræa Centaurium，现代名称则为 Centaurium umbellatum。

续表

| 英文名 | 拉丁名 ① （植物学名称） | 现有翻译 | 本书翻译 |
|---|---|---|---|
| Crab Apple | Malus pumila | 海棠、山楂、西洋苹果、野生酸苹果 | 野生酸苹果 |
| Elm | Ulmus procera | 榆树 | 榆树 |
| Gentian | Gentiana amarelle | 龙胆、龙胆根、龙胆草 | 龙胆 |
| Gorse | Ulex europaeus | 荆豆、金雀花 | 荆豆 |
| Heather | Calluna vulgaris | 石南、石楠 | 石楠 |
| Holly | Ilex aquifolium | 冬青 | 冬青 |
| Honeysuckle | Lonicera caprifolium | 忍冬 | 忍冬 |
| Hornbeam | Carpinus betulus | 鹅耳枥、铁树 | 鹅耳枥 |
| Impatiens | Impatiens glandulifera | 凤仙花 | 凤仙花 |
| Larch | Larix decidua | 落叶松 | 落叶松 |
| Mimulus | Mimulus guttatus | 龙头花、沟酸浆、构酸酱 | 构酸酱 |
| Mustard | Sinapis arvensis | 芥茉、芥子 | 芥末 |
| Oak | Quercus robur | 橡树 | 橡树 |
| Olive | Olea europaea | 橄榄 | 橄榄 |
| Pine | Pinus sylvestris | 松树、欧洲赤松、松针 | 松针 |
| Red Chestnut | Aesculus carnea | 红栗、红栗子、红西洋栗、红栗花 | 红西洋栗 |
| Rock Rose | Helianthemum nummularium | 岩蔷薇 | 岩蔷薇 |
| Scleranthus | Scleranthus annuus | 线球草、史开兰、硬花草 | 线球草 |

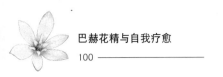

续表

| 英文名 | 拉丁名①（植物学名称） | 现有翻译 | 本书翻译 |
|---|---|---|---|
| Star of Bethlehem | Ornithogalum umbellatum | 伯利恒之星、圣星百合 | 圣星百合 |
| Sweet Chestnut | Castanea sativa | 甜西洋栗、甜栗子、西洋栗、甜栗花 | 甜西洋栗 |
| Vervain | Verbena officinalis | 马鞭草 | 马鞭草 |
| Vine | Vitis Vinifera | 葡萄藤、葡萄 | 葡萄树 |
| Walnut | Juglans regia | 胡桃、核桃 | 胡桃 |
| Water Violet | Hottonia palustris | 水堇、水紫、美洲赫顿草 | 水堇 |
| White Chestnut | Aesculus hippocastanum | 白栗花、白栗子 | 白栗花 |
| Wild Oat | Bromus ramosus Bromus Asper | 野燕麦、野生燕麦 | 野生燕麦 |
| Wild Rose | Rosa canina | 野玫瑰、野蔷薇 | 野玫瑰 |
| Willow | Salix vitellina | 柳树、柳树、黄柳 | 柳树 |
| Rock Water | | 岩泉水、岩清水、岩水 | 岩泉水 |

巴赫医生的中文译名还有巴哈、贝曲、贝齐，巴赫花精的中文译名还有巴哈花药、巴哈花精、贝曲花精。

附录2

# 第一部英文版
## *Heal Thyself*

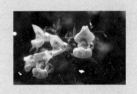

# HEAL
# THYSELF

An explanation of the real cause and cure of disease

## EDWARD BACH

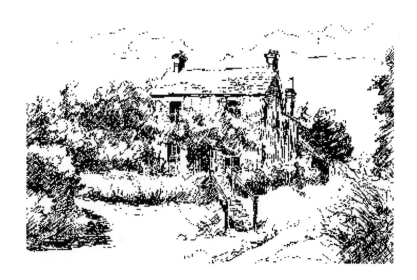

This book is dedicated

to all who suffer or who are in distress.

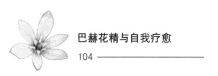
# FOREWORD

Edward Bach wrote *Heal Thyself* in 1930, in Abersoch, Wales. The original title of the book was to be *Come Out into the Sunshine* - and from Lord Buddha's appearance in chapter one right through to that of the "White Brotherhood" of the spiritually aware in the final paragraph, the idea of bringing light to all of humanity is a constant thread.

Bach had left London a few months before to dedicate himself to his emerging system of flower healing, and had only just discovered the sun method of remedy preparation. By the time he completed his research a few years later some of the ideas in *Heal Thyself* had already gone out of date. The links suggested in chapter three between specific physical symptoms and named emotions proved unreliable when it came to selecting flower remedies and were abandoned. His ideas about "the physician of the future" had been aimed at doctors and not their patients; by 1932 he had realised that now, thanks to the remedies, "we are all healers".

But the core of the book remains relevant to all modern practitioners and users of the Bach flower remedies. *Heal Thyself* represents Bach's views on medicine, spirituality, health and healing. Many of its key concepts were crucial in guiding his research. It is significant that of all his writings it was this book, along with *The Twelve Healers and Other Remedies*, that he most wanted to survive.

Stefan Ball

The Bach Centre

November 2013

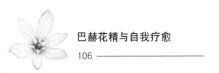
# CHAPTER ONE

It is not the object of this book to suggest that the art of healing is unnecessary; far be from it any such intention; but it is humbly hoped that it will be a guide to those who suffer to seek within themselves the real origin of their maladies, so that they may assist themselves in their own healing. Moreover, it is hoped that it may stimulate those, both in the medical profession and in religious orders, who have the welfare of humanity at heart, to redouble their efforts in seeking the relief of human suffering, and so hasten that day when the victory over disease will be complete.

The main reason for the failure of modern medical science is that it is dealing with results and not causes. For many centuries the real nature of disease has been masked by materialism, and thus disease itself has been given every opportunity of extending its ravages, since it has not been attacked at its origin. The situation is like to an enemy strongly fortified in the hills, continually waging guerrilla warfare in the country around, while the people, ignoring the fortified garrison, content themselves with repairing the damaged houses and burying the dead, which are the result of the raids of the marauders. So, generally speaking, is the situation in medicine today; nothing more than the patching up of those attacked and the burying of those who are slain, without a thought being given to the real stronghold.

Disease will never be cured or eradicated by present materialistic methods, for the simple reason that disease in its origin is not material. What we know as disease is an ultimate result produced in the body, the end product of deep and long acting forces, and even if material treatment alone is apparently successful this is nothing more than a temporary relief unless the real cause has been removed. The modern trend of medical science, by misinterpreting the true nature of disease and concentrating it in materialistic terms in the physical body, has enormously increased its power, firstly, by distracting the thoughts of people from its true origin and hence from the effective method of attack, and secondly, by localising it in the body, thus obscuring true hope of recovery and raising a mighty disease complex of fear, which never should have existed.

Disease is in essence the result of conflict between Soul and Mind, and will never be eradicated except by spiritual and mental effort. Such efforts, if properly made with understanding as we shall see later, can cure and prevent disease by removing those basic factors which are its primary cause. No effort directed to the body alone can do more than superficially repair damage, and in this there is no cure, since the cause is still operative and may at any moment again demonstrate its presence in another form. In fact, in many cases apparent recovery is harmful, since it hides from the patient the true cause of his trouble, and in the satisfaction of apparently renewed health the real factor, being unnoticed, may gain in strength. Contrast these cases with that of the patient who knows, or who is by some wise physician instructed in, the nature of the adverse spiritual or mental forces at work, the result of which has precipitated what we call disease in the physical body. If that patient directly attempts to neutralise those forces, health improves as soon as this is successfully begun, and when it is completed the disease will disappear. This is true healing by attacking the stronghold, the very base of the cause of suffering.

One of the exceptions to materialistic methods in modern science is that of the great Hahnemann, the founder of Homeopathy, who with his realisation of the beneficent love of the Creator and of the Divinity which resides within man, by studying the mental attitude of his patients towards life, environment and their respective diseases, sought to find in the herbs of the field and in the realms of nature the remedy which would not only heal their bodies but would at the same time uplift their mental outlook. May his science be extended and developed by those true physicians who have the love of humanity at heart.

Five hundred years before Christ some physicians of ancient India, working under the influence of the Lord Buddha, advanced the art of healing to so perfect a state that they were able to abolish surgery, although the surgery of their time was as efficient, or more so, than that of the present day. Such men as Hippocrates with his mighty ideals of healing, Paracelsus with his certainty of the divinity in man, and Hahnemann who realised that disease originated in a plane above the physical – all these knew much of the real nature and remedy of suffering. What untold misery would have been spared during the last twenty or twenty-five centuries had the teaching of these great masters of their art been followed, but, as in other things, materialism has appealed too strongly to the Western world, and for so long a time, that the voices of the practical obstructors have risen above the advice of those who knew the truth.

Let it be briefly stated that disease, though apparently so cruel, is in itself beneficent and for our good and, if rightly interpreted, it will guide us to our essential faults. If properly treated it will be the cause of the removal of those faults and leave us better and greater than before. Suffering is a corrective to point out a lesson which by other means we have failed to grasp, and never can it be eradicated until that lesson is learnt. Let it also be known that in those who understand and are able to read the significance of premonitory symptoms disease may be prevented before its onset or aborted in its earlier stages if the proper corrective spiritual and mental efforts be undertaken. Nor need any case despair, however severe, for the fact that the individual is still granted physical life indicates that the Soul who rules is not without hope.

# CHAPTER TWO

To understand the nature of disease certain fundamental truths have to be acknowledged.

The first of these is that man has a Soul which is his real self; a Divine, Mighty Being, a Son of the Creator of all things, of which the body, although the earthly temple of that Soul, is but the minutest reflection: that our Soul, our Divinity Who resides in and around us, lays down for us our lives as He wishes them to be ordered and, so far as we will allow, ever guides, protects and encourages us, watchful and beneficent to lead us always for our utmost advantage: that He, our Higher Self, being a spark of the Almighty, is thereby invincible and immortal.

The second principle is that we, as we know ourselves in this world, are personalities down here for the purpose of gaining all the knowledge and experience which can be obtained through earthly existence, of developing virtues which we lack and of wiping out all that is wrong within us, thus advancing towards the perfection of our natures. The Soul knows what environment and what circumstances will best enable us to do this, and hence He places us in that branch of life most suited for that object.

Thirdly, we must realise that the short passage on this earth, which we know as life, is but a moment in the course of our evolution, as one day at school is to a life, and although we can for the present only see and comprehend that one day, our intuition tells us that birth was infinitely far from our beginning and death infinitely far from our ending. Our Souls, which are really we, are immortal, and the bodies of which we are conscious are temporary, merely as horses we ride to go a journey, or instruments we use to do a piece of work.

Then follows a fourth great principle, that so long as our Souls and personalities are in harmony all is joy and peace, happiness and health. It is when our personalities are led astray from the path laid down by the Soul, either by our own worldly desires or by the persuasion of others, that a conflict arises. This conflict is the root cause of disease and unhappiness. No matter what our work in the world – bootblack or monarch, landlord or peasant, rich or poor – so long as we do that particular work according to the dictates of the Soul, all is well; and we can further rest assured that in whatever station of life we are placed, princely or lowly, it contains the lessons and experiences necessary at the moment for our evolution, and gives us the best advantage for the development of ourselves.

The next great principle is the understanding of the Unity of all things: that the Creator of all things is Love, and that everything of which we are conscious is in all its infinite number of forms a manifestation of that Love, whether it be a planet or a pebble, a star or a dewdrop, man or the lowliest form of life. It may be possible to get a glimpse of this conception by thinking of our Creator as a great blazing sun of beneficence and love and from the centre an infinite number of beams radiate in every direction, and that we and all of which we are conscious are particles at the end of those beams, sent out to gain experience and knowledge, but ultimately to return to the great centre. And though to us each ray may appear separate and distinct, it is in reality part of the great central Sun. Separation is impossible, for as soon as a beam of light is cut off from its source it ceases to exist. Thus we may comprehend a little of the impossibility of separateness, as although each ray may have its individuality, it is nevertheless part of the great central creative power. Thus any action against ourselves or against another affects the whole, because by causing imperfection in a part it reflects on the whole, every particle of which must ultimately become perfect.

So we see there are two great possible fundamental errors: dissociation between our Souls and our personalities, and cruelty or wrong to others, for this is a sin against Unity. Either of these brings conflict, which leads to disease. An understanding of where we are making an error (which is so often not realised by us) and an earnest endeavour to correct the fault will lead not only to a life of joy and peace, but also to health.

Disease is in itself beneficent, and has for its object the bringing back of the personality to the Divine will of the Soul; and thus we can see that it is both preventable and avoidable, since if we could only realise for ourselves the mistakes we are making and correct these by spiritual and mental means there could be no need for the severe lessons of suffering. Every opportunity is given us by the Divine Power to mend our ways before, as a last resort, pain and suffering have to be applied. It may not be the errors of this life, this day at school, which we are combating; and although we in our physical minds may not be conscious of the reason of our suffering, which may to us appear cruel and without reason, yet our Souls (which are ourselves) know the full purpose and are guiding us to our best advantage. Nevertheless, understanding and correction of our errors would shorten our illness and bring us back to health. Knowledge of the Soul's purpose and acquiescence in that knowledge means the relief of earthly suffering and distress, and leaves us free to develop our evolution in joy and happiness.

There are two great errors: first, to fail to honour and obey the dictates of our Soul, and second, to act against Unity. On account of the former, be ever reluctant to judge others, because what is right for one is wrong for another. The merchant, whose work it is to build up a big trade not only to his own advantage but also to that of all those whom he may employ, thereby gaining knowledge of efficiency and control and developing the virtues associated with each, must of necessity use different qualities and different virtues from those of a nurse, sacrificing her life in the care of the sick; and yet both, if obeying the dictates of their Souls, are rightly learning those qualities necessary for their evolution. It is obeying the commands of

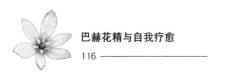
our Soul, our Higher Self, which we learn through conscience, instinct and intuition, that matters.

Thus we see that by its very principles and in its very essence, disease is both preventable and curable, and it is the work of spiritual healers and physicians to give, in addition to material remedies, the knowledge to the suffering of the error of their lives, and of the manner in which these errors can be eradicated, and so to lead the sick back to health and joy.

# CHAPTER THREE

What we know as disease is the terminal stage of a much deeper disorder, and to ensure complete success in treatment it is obvious that dealing with the final result alone will not be wholly effective unless the basic cause is also removed. There is one primary error which man can make, and that is action against Unity; this originates in self-love. So also we may say that there is but one primary affliction – discomfort, or disease. And as action against Unity may be divided into various types, so also may disease – the result of these actions – be separated into main groups corresponding to their causes. The very nature of an illness will be a useful guide to assist in discovering the type of action which is being taken against the Divine Law of Love and Unity.

If we have in our nature sufficient love of all things, then we can do no harm; because that love would stay our hand at any action, our mind at any thought which might hurt another.

But we have not yet reached that state of perfection; if we had, there would be no need for our existence here. But all of us are seeking and advancing towards that state, and those of us who suffer in mind or body are by this very suffering being led towards that ideal condition; and if we will but read it aright, we may not only hasten our steps towards that goal, but also save ourselves illness and distress. From the moment the lesson is understood and the error eliminated there is no longer need for the correction, because we must remember that suffering is in itself beneficent, in that it points out to us when we are taking wrong paths and hastens our evolution to its glorious perfection.

The real primary diseases of man are such defects as pride, cruelty, hate, self-love, ignorance, instability and greed; and each of these, if considered, will be found to be adverse to Unity. Such defects as these are the real diseases (using the word in the modern sense), and it is a continuation and persistence in such defects after we have reached that stage of development when we know them to be wrong, which precipitates in the body the injurious results which we know as illness.

Pride is due, firstly, to lack of recognition of the smallness of the personality and its utter dependence on the Soul, and that all the successes it may have are not of itself but are blessings bestowed by the Divinity within; secondly, the loss of the sense of proportion, of the minuteness of one amidst the scheme of Creation. As Pride invariably refuses to bend with humility and resignation to the Will of the Great Creator, it commits actions contrary to that Will.

Cruelty is a denial of the unity of all and a failure to understand that any action adverse to another is in opposition to the whole, and hence an action against Unity. No man would practise its injurious effects against those near and dear to him, and by the law of Unity we have to grow until we understand that everyone, as being part of a whole, must become near and dear to us, until even those who persecute us call up only feelings of love and sympathy.

Hate is the opposite of Love, the reverse of the Law of Creation. It is contrary to the whole Divine scheme and is a denial of the Creator; it leads only to such actions and thoughts which are adverse to Unity and the opposite of those which would be dictated by Love.

Self-love again is a denial of Unity and the duty we owe

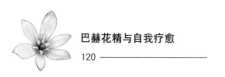
to our brother men by putting the interests of ourselves before the good of humanity and the care and protection of those immediately around us.

Ignorance is the failure to learn, the refusal to see Truth when the opportunity is offered, and leads to many wrong acts such as can only exist in darkness and are not possible when the light of Truth and Knowledge is around us.

Instability, indecision and weakness of purpose result when the personality refuses to be ruled by the Higher Self, and lead us to betray others through our weakness. Such a condition would not be possible had we within us the knowledge of the Unconquerable Invincible Divinity which is in reality ourselves.

Greed leads to a desire for power. It is a denial of the freedom and individuality of every soul. Instead of recognising that every one of us is down here to develop freely upon his own lines according to the dictates of the soul alone, to increase his individuality, and to work free and unhampered, the personality with greed desires to dictate, mould and command, usurping the power of the Creator.

Such are examples of real disease, the origin and basis of all our suffering and distress. Each of such defects, if persisted in against the voice of the Higher Self, will produce a conflict which must of necessity be reflected in the physical body, producing its own specific type of malady.

We can now see how any type of illness from which we may suffer will guide us to the discovery of the fault which lies behind our affliction. [1] For example, Pride, which is arrogance and rigidity of mind, will give rise to those diseases which produce rigidity and stiffness of the body. Pain is the result of cruelty, whereby the patient learns through personal suffering not to inflict it upon others, either from a physical or from a mental standpoint. The penalties of Hate are loneliness, violent uncontrollable temper, mental nerve storms and conditions of hysteria. The diseases of introspection – neurosis, neurasthenia and similar conditions – which rob life of so much enjoyment, are caused by excessive Self-love. Ignorance and lack of wisdom bring their own difficulties in everyday life, and in addition should there be a persistence in refusing to see truth when the opportunity has been given, short-sightedness and impairment of vision and hearing are the natural consequences.

———————————

[1]　See the *Foreword*, page 4

Instability of mind must lead to the same quality in the body with those various disorders which affect movement and co-ordination. The result of greed and domination of others is such diseases as will render the sufferer a slave to his own body, with desires and ambitions curbed by the malady.

Moreover, the very part of the body affected is no accident, but is in accordance with the law of cause and effect, and again will be a guide to help us. For example, the heart, the fountain of life and hence of love, is attacked when especially the love side of the nature towards humanity is not developed or is wrongly used; a hand affected denotes failure or wrong in action; the brain being the centre of control, if afflicted, indicates lack of control in the personality. Such must follow as the law lays down. We are all ready to admit the many results which may follow a fit of violent temper, the shock of sudden bad news; if trivial affairs can thus affect the body, how much more serious and deep-rooted must be a prolonged conflict between soul and body. Can we wonder that the result gives rise to such grievous complaints as the diseases amongst us today?

But yet there is no cause for depression. The prevention and cure of disease can be found by discovering the wrong within ourselves and eradicating this fault by the earnest development of the virtue which will destroy it; not by fighting the wrong, but by bringing in such a flood of its opposing virtue that it will be swept from our natures.

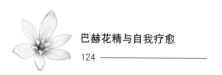

# CHAPTER FOUR

So we find that there is nothing of the nature of accident as regards disease, either in its type or in that part of the body which is affected; like all other results of energy, it follows the law of cause and effect. Certain maladies may be caused by direct physical means, such as those associated with some poisons, accidents and injuries, and gross excesses; but disease in general is due to some basic error in our constitution, as in the examples already given.

And thus for a complete cure not only must physical means be used, choosing always the best methods which are known to the art of healing, but we ourselves must also endeavour to the utmost of our ability to remove any fault in our nature; because final and complete healing ultimately comes from within, from the Soul itself, which by His beneficence radiates harmony throughout the personality, when allowed to do so.

As there is one great root cause of all disease, namely

self-love, so there is one great certain method of relief of all suffering, the conversion of self-love into devotion to others. If we but sufficiently develop the quality of losing ourselves in the love and care of those around us, enjoying the glorious adventure of gaining knowledge and helping others, our personal griefs and sufferings rapidly come to an end. It is the great ultimate aim: the losing of our own interests in the service of humanity. It matters not the station in life in which our Divinity has placed us. Whether engaged in trade or profession, rich or poor, monarch or beggar, for one and all it is possible to carry on the work of their respective vocations and yet be veritable blessings to those around by communicating to them the Divine Love of Brotherhood.

But the vast majority of us have some way to travel before we can reach this state of perfection, although it is surprising how rapidly any individual may advance along these lines if the effort is seriously made, providing he trusts not in his poor personality alone but has implicit faith, that by the example and teaching of the great masters of the world he may be enabled to unite himself with his own Soul, the Divinity within, when all things become possible. In most of us there is one, or more, adverse defect which is particularly hindering our advancement, and it is such defect, or defects, which we must especially seek out within ourselves, and whilst striving to develop and extend the love side of our nature towards the world, endeavour at the same time to wash away any such defect in particular by the flooding of our nature with the opposing virtue. At first this may be a little difficult, but only just at first, for it is remarkable how rapidly a truly encouraged virtue will increase, linked with the knowledge that with the aid of the Divinity within us, if we but persevere, failure is impossible.

In the development of Universal Love within ourselves we must learn to realise more and more that every human being, however lowly, is a son of the Creator, and that one day and in due time he will advance to perfection just as we all hope to do. However base a man or creature may appear, we must remember that there is the Divine Spark within, which will slowly but surely grow until the glory of the Creator irradiates that being.

Moreover, the question of right or wrong, of good and evil, is purely relative. That which is right in the natural evolution of the aboriginal would be wrong for the more enlightened of our civilisation, and that which might even be a virtue in such as ourselves might be out of place, and hence wrong, in one who has reached the stage of discipleship. What we call wrong or evil is in reality good out of place, and hence is purely relative. Let us remember also that our standard of idealism again is relative; to the animals we must appear as veritable gods, whereas we in ourselves are very far below the standards of the great White Brotherhood[①] of Saints and Martyrs who have given their all to be examples to us. Hence we must have compassion and sympathy for the lowliest, for whilst we may consider ourselves as having advanced far above their level, we are in ourselves minute indeed, and have yet a long journey before us to reach the standard of our older brothers, whose light shines throughout the world in every age.

If Pride assails us, let us try to realise that our personalities are in themselves as nothing, unable to do any good work or acceptable service, or to resist the powers of darkness, unless assisted by that Light which is from above, the Light of our Soul; endeavour to comprehend a glimpse of the omnipotence

---

① See the *Foreword*, page 4

and unthinkable mightiness of our Creator, Who makes in all perfection a world in one drop of water and systems upon systems of universes, and try to realise the relative humility we owe and our utter dependence upon Him. We learn to pay homage and give respect to our human superiors; how infinitely more should we acknowledge our own frailty with utmost humility before the Great Architect of the Universe!

If Cruelty, or Hate, bar our way to progress, let us remember that Love is the foundation of Creation, that in every living soul there is some good, and that in the best of us there is some bad. By seeking the good in others, even in those who at first offend us, we shall learn to develop, if nothing more, some sympathy and a hope that they will see better ways; then it follows that the desire will arise to help them to that uplift. The ultimate conquest of all will be through love and gentleness, and when we have sufficiently developed these two qualities nothing will be able to assail us, since we shall ever have compassion and not offer resistance; for, again, by the same law of cause and effect it is resistance which damages. Our object in life is to follow the dictates of our Higher Self, undeterred by the influence of others, and this can only be achieved if we gently go our own way, but at the same time never interfere with the personality of another or cause the least harm by any method of cruelty or hate. We must strive to learn love of others, beginning perhaps with one individual or even an animal, and let this love develop and extend over a wider and wider range, until its opposing defects will automatically disappear. Love begets Love, as Hate does Hate.

The cure of self-love is effected by the turning outwards to others of the care and attention which we are devoting to ourselves, becoming so engrossed in their welfare that we forget ourselves in that endeavour. As one great order of Brotherhood expresses it, "to seek the solace of our own distress by extending relief and consolation to our fellowcreatures in the hour of their affliction," and there is no surer way of curing self-love and the disorders which follow it than by such a method.

Instability can be eradicated by the development of self-determination, by making up the mind and doing things with definiteness instead of wavering and hovering. Even if at first we may sometimes make errors, it were better to act than to let opportunities pass for the want of decision. Determination will soon grow; fear of plunging into life will disappear, and the experiences gained will guide our mind to better judgement.

To eradicate Ignorance, again let us not be afraid of experience, but with mind awake and with eyes and ears wide open take in every particle of knowledge which may be obtained. At the same time we must keep flexible in thought, lest preconceived ideas and former convictions rob us of the opportunity of gaining fresh and wider knowledge. We should be ever ready to expand the mind and to disregard any idea, however firmly rooted, if under wider experience a greater truth shows itself.

Like Pride, Greed is a great obstacle to advancement, and both of these must be ruthlessly washed away. The results of Greed are serious indeed, because it leads us to interfere with the souldevelopment of our fellow-men. We must realise that every being is here to develop his own evolution according to the dictates of his Soul, and his Soul alone, and that none of us must do anything but encourage our brother in that development. We must help him to hope and, if in our power, increase his knowledge and worldly opportunities to gain his advancement. Just as we would wish others to help us up the steep and difficult mountain path of life, so let us be ever ready to lend a helping hand and give the experience of our wider knowledge to a weaker or younger brother. Such should be the attitude of parent to child, master to man or comrade to comrade, giving care, love and protection as far as may be needed and beneficial, yet never for one moment interfering with the natural evolution of the personality, as this must be dictated by the Soul.

Many of us in our childhood and early life are much nearer to our own Soul than we are in later years, and have then clearer ideas of our work in life, the endeavours we are expected to make and the character we are required to develop. The reason for this is that the materialism and circumstances of our age, and the personalities with whom we associate, lead us away from the voice of our Higher Self and bind us firmly to the commonplace with its lack of ideals, all too evident in this civilisation. Let the parent, the master and the comrade ever strive to encourage the growth of the Higher Self within those over whom they have the wonderful privilege and opportunity to exert their influence, but let them ever allow freedom to others, as they hope to have freedom given to them.

So in a similar way may we seek out any faults in our constitution and wash them out by developing the opposing virtue, thus removing from our nature the cause of the conflict between Soul and personality, which is the primary basic cause of disease. Such action alone, if the patient has faith and strength, will bring relief, health and joy, and in those not so strong will materially assist the work of the earthly physician in bringing about the same result.

We must earnestly learn to develop individuality according to the dictates of our own Soul, to fear no man and to see that no one interferes with, or dissuades us from, the development of our evolution, the fulfilment of our duty and the rendering of help to our fellow-men, remembering that the further we advance, the greater blessing we become to those around. Especially must we be on guard in the giving of help to other people, no matter whom they be, to be certain that the desire to help comes from the dictates of the Inner Self and is not a false sense of duty imposed by the suggestion or persuasion of a more dominant personality. One tragedy resulting from modern convention is of such a type, and it is impossible to calculate the thousands of hindered lives, the myriads of missed opportunities, the sorrow and the suffering so caused, the countless number of children who from a sense of duty have perhaps for years waited upon an invalid when the only malady the parent has known has been the greed of attention. Think of the armies of men and women who have been prevented from doing perhaps some great and useful work for humanity because their personality has been captured by some one individual from whom they have not had the courage to win freedom; the children who in their early days know and desire their ordained calling, and yet from difficulties of circumstance, dissuasion by others and weakness of purpose glide into some other branch of life, where they are neither happy nor able to develop their evolution as they might otherwise have done. It is the dictates of our conscience alone which can tell us whether our duty lies with one or many, how and whom we should serve; but whichever it may be, we should obey that command to the utmost of our ability.

Finally, let us not fear to plunge into life; we are here to gain experience and knowledge, and we shall learn but little unless we face realities and seek to our utmost. Such experience can be gained in every quarter, and the truths of nature and of humanity can be won just as effectively, perhaps even more so, in a country cottage as amongst the noise and hustle of a city.

# CHAPTER FIVE

As lack of individuality (that is, the allowing of interference with the personality, such interference preventing it from complying with the demands of the Higher Self) is of such great importance in the production of disease, and as it often begins early in life, let us now consider the true relation between parent and child, teacher and pupil.

Fundamentally, the office of parenthood is to be the privileged means (and, indeed, it should be considered as divinely privileged) of enabling a soul to contact this world for the sake of evolution. If properly understood, there is probably no greater opportunity offered to mankind than this, to be the agent of the physical birth of a soul and to have the care of the young personality during the first few years of its existence on earth. The whole attitude of parents should be to give the little newcomer all the spiritual, mental and physical guidance to the utmost of their ability, ever remembering that the wee one is an individual soul come down to gain his own experience and knowledge in his own way according to the dictates of his Higher Self, and every possible freedom should be given for unhampered development.

The office of parenthood is one of divine service, and should be respected as much as, or perhaps even more than, any other duty we may be called upon to undertake. As it is one of sacrifice, it must ever be borne in mind that nothing whatever should be required in return from the child, the whole object being to give, and give alone, gentle love, protection and guidance until the soul takes charge of the young personality. Independence, individuality and freedom, should be taught from the beginning, and the child should be encouraged as early as possible in life to think and act for himself. All parental control should be relinquished step by step as the ability for selfmanagement is developed, and later on no restraint or false idea of duty to parenthood should hamper the dictates of the child's soul.

Parenthood is an office in life which passes from one to another, and is in essence a temporary giving of guidance and protection for a brief period, after which time it should then cease its efforts and leave the object of its attention free to advance alone. Be it remembered that the child for whom we may become a temporary guardian may be a much older and greater soul than ourselves, and spiritually our superior, so that control and protection should be confined to the needs of the young personality.

Parenthood is a sacred duty, temporary in its character and passing from generation to generation. It carries with it nothing but service and calls for no obligation in return from the young, since they must be left free to develop in their own way and become as fitted as possible to fulfil the same office in but a few years' time. Thus the child should have no restrictions, no obligations and no parental hindrances, knowing that parenthood had previously been bestowed on his father and mother and that it may be his duty to perform the same office for another.

Parents should be particularly on guard against any desire to mould the young personality according to their own ideas or wishes, and should refrain from any undue control or demand of favours in return for their natural duty and divine privilege of being the means of helping a soul to contact the world. Any desire for control, or wish to shape the young life for personal motives, is a terrible form of greed and should never be countenanced, for if in the young father or mother this takes root it will in later years lead them to be veritable vampires. If there is the least desire to dominate, it should be checked at the onset. We must refuse to be under the slavery of greed, which compels in us the wish to possess others. We must encourage in ourselves the art of giving, and develop this until it has washed out by its sacrifice every trace of adverse action.

The teacher should ever bear in mind that it is his office merely to be the agent of giving to the young guidance and an opportunity of learning the things of the world and of life, so that each child may absorb knowledge in his own way, and, if allowed freedom, instinctively choose that which is necessary for the success of his life. Again, therefore, nothing more than the gentlest care and guidance should be given to enable the student to gain the knowledge he requires.

Children should remember that the office of parenthood, as emblematical of creative power, is divine in its mission, but that it calls for no restriction of development and no obligations which might hamper the life and work dictated to them by their own Soul. It is impossible to estimate in this present civilisation the untold suffering, the cramping of natures and the developing of dominant characters which the lack of a realisation of this fact produces. In almost every home parents and children build themselves prisons from entirely false motives and a wrong conception of the relationship of parent and child. These prisons bar the freedom, cramp the life, prevent the natural development and bring unhappiness to all concerned, and the mental, nervous and even physical disorders which afflict such people form a very large proportion indeed of the sickness of our present time.

It cannot be too firmly realised that every soul in incarnation is down here for the specific purpose of gaining experience and understanding, and of perfecting his personality towards those ideals laid down by the soul. No matter what our relationship be to each other, whether husband and wife, parent and child, brother and sister, or master and man, we sin against our Creator and against our fellow-men if we hinder from motives of personal desire the evolution of another soul. Our sole duty is to obey the dictates of our own conscience, and this will never for one moment brook the domination of another personality. Let everyone remember that his Soul has laid down for him a particular work, and that unless he does this work, though perhaps not consciously, he will inevitably raise a conflict between his Soul and personality which of necessity reacts in the form of physical disorders.

True, it may be the calling of any one individual to devote his life to one other alone, but before doing so let him be absolutely certain that this is the command of his Soul, and that it is not the suggestion of some other dominant personality over-persuading him, or false ideas of duty misdirecting him. Let him also remember that we come down into this world to win battles, to gain strength against those who would control us, and to advance to that stage when we pass through life doing our duty quietly and calmly, undeterred and uninfluenced by any living being, calmly guided always by the voice of our Higher Self. For very many their greatest battle will be in their own home, where before gaining their liberty to win victories in the world they will have to free themselves from the adverse domination and control of some very near relative.

Any individual, whether adult or child, part of whose work it is in this life to free himself from the dominant control of another, should remember the following: firstly, that his would-be oppressor should be regarded in the same way as we look upon an opponent in sport, as a personality with whom we are playing the game of Life, without the least trace of bitterness, and that if it were not for such opponents we should be lacking the opportunity of developing our own courage and individuality; secondly, that the real victories of life come through love and gentleness, and that in such a contest no force whatever must be used: that by steadily growing in his own nature, bearing sympathy, kindness and, if possible, affection – or, even better, love – towards the opponent, he may so develop that in time he may very gently and quietly follow the call of conscience without allowing the least interference.

Those who are dominant require much help and guidance to enable them to realise the great universal truth of Unity and to understand the joy of Brotherhood. To miss such things is to miss the real happiness of Life, and we must help such folk as far as lies within our power. Weakness on our part, which allows them to extend their influence, will in no way assist them; a gentle refusal to be under their control and an endeavour to bring to them the realisation of the joy of giving will help them along the upward path.

The gaining of our freedom, the winning of our

individuality and independence, will in most cases call for much courage and faith. But in the darkest hours, and when success seems well-nigh impossible, let us ever remember that God's children should never be afraid, that our Souls only give us such tasks as we are capable of accomplishing, and that with our own courage and faith in the Divinity within us victory must come to all who continue to strive.

# CHAPTER SIX

And now, dear brothers and sisters, when we realise that Love and Unity are the great foundations of our Creation, that we in ourselves are children of the Divine Love, and that the eternal conquest of all wrong and suffering will be accomplished by means of gentleness and love, when we realise all this, where in this beauteous picture are we to place such practices as vivisection and animal gland grafting? Are we still so primitive, so pagan, that we yet believe that by the sacrifice of animals we are enabled to escape the results of our own faults and failings? Nearly 2,500 years ago the Lord Buddha showed to the world the wrongness of sacrificing the lower creatures. Humanity already owes a mighty debt to the animals which it has tortured and destroyed, and far from any good resulting to man from such inhuman practices, nothing but harm and damage can be wrought to both the human and animal kingdoms. How far have we of the West wandered from those beautiful ideals of our

Mother India of old times, when so great was the love for the creatures of the earth that men were trained and skilled to attend the maladies and injuries of not only the animals, but also the birds. Moreover, there were vast sanctuaries for all types of life, and so averse were the people to hurting a lower creature that any man who hunted was refused the attendance of a physician in time of sickness until he had vowed to relinquish such a practice.

Let us not speak against the men who practise vivisection, for numbers of these are working with truly humanitarian principles, hoping and striving to find some relief for human suffering; their motive is good enough, but their wisdom is poor, and they have little understanding of the reason of life. Motive alone, however right, is not enough; it must be combined with wisdom and knowledge.

Of the horror of the black magic associated with gland grafting let us not even write, but implore every human being to shun it as ten thousand times worse than any plague, for it is a sin against God, man and animal.

With just such one or two exceptions there is no point in dwelling on the failure of modern medical science; destruction is useless unless we rebuild a better edifice, and as in medicine the foundation of the newer building is already laid, let us concentrate on adding one or two stones to that temple. Neither is adverse criticism of the profession to-day of value; it is the system which is mainly wrong, not the men; for it is a system whereby the physician, from economic reasons alone, has not the time for administering quiet, peaceful treatment or the opportunity for the necessary meditation and thought which should be the heritage of those who devote their lives to attendance on the sick. As Paracelsus said, the wise physician attends five, not fifteen, patients in a day – an ideal impracticable in this age for the average practitioner.

The dawn of a new and better art of healing is upon us. A hundred years ago the Homeopathy of Hahnemann was as the first streak of the morning light after a long night of darkness, and it may play a big part in the medicine of the future. Moreover, the attention which is being given at the present time to improving conditions of life and providing purer and cleaner diet is an advance towards the prevention of sickness; and those movements which are directed to bring to the notice of the people both the connection between spiritual failings and disease and the healing which may be obtained through perfection of the mind, are pointing the way towards the coming of that bright sunshine in whose radiant light the darkness of disease will disappear.

Let us remember that disease is a common enemy, and that every one of us who conquers a fragment of it is thereby helping not only himself but the whole of humanity. A certain, but definite, amount of energy will have to be expended before its overthrow is complete; let us one and all strive for this result, and those who are greater and stronger than the others may not only do their share, but materially assist their weaker brothers.

Obviously the first way to prevent the spread and increase of disease is for us to cease committing those actions which extend its power; the second, to wipe out from our natures our own defects, which would allow further invasion. The achievement of this is victory indeed; then, having freed ourselves, we are free to help others. And it is not so difficult as it may at first appear; we are but expected to do our best, and we know that this is possible for all of us if we will but listen to the dictates of our own Soul. Life does not demand of us unthinkable sacrifice; it asks us to travel its journey with joy in our heart and to be a blessing to those around, so that if we leave the world just that trifle better for our visit, then have we done our work.

The teachings of religions, if properly read, plead with us "to forsake all and follow Me", the interpretation of which is to give ourselves entirely up to the demands of our Higher Self, but not, as some imagine, to discard home and comfort, love and luxury; very far from this is the truth. A prince of the realm, with all the glories of the palace, may be a Godsend and a blessing indeed to his people, to his country – nay, even to the world; how much might have been lost had that prince imagined it his duty to enter a monastery. The offices of life in every branch, from the lowliest to the most exalted, have to be filled, and the Divine Guide of our destinies knows into which office to place us for our best advantage; all we are expected to do is to fulfil that duty cheerfully and well. There are saints at the factory bench and in the stokehold of a ship as well as among the dignitaries of religious orders. Not one of us upon this earth is being asked to do more than is within his power to perform, and if we strive to obtain the best within us, ever guided by our Higher Self, health and happiness is a possibility for each one.

For the greater part of the last two thousand years Western civilisation has passed through an age of intense materialism, and the realisation of the spiritual side of our natures and existence has been greatly lost in the attitude of mind which has placed worldly possessions, ambitions, desires and pleasures above the real things of life. The true reason of man's existence on earth has been overshadowed by his anxiety to obtain from his incarnation nothing but worldly gain. It has been a period when life has been very difficult because of the lack of the real comfort, encouragement and uplift which is brought by a realisation of greater things than those of the world. During the last centuries religions have to many people appeared rather as legends having no bearing on their lives instead of being the very essence of their existence. The true nature of our Higher Self, the knowledge of previous and later life, apart from this present one, has meant but very little to us instead of being the guide and stimulus of our every action. We have rather shunned the great things and attempted to make life as comfortable as possible by putting the super-physical out of our minds and depending upon earthly pleasures to compensate us for our trials. Thus have position, rank, wealth and worldly possessions become the goal of these centuries; and as all such things are transient and can only be obtained and held with much anxiety and concentration on material things, so has the real internal peace and happiness of the past generations been infinitely below that which is the due of mankind.

The real peace of the Soul and mind is with us when we are making spiritual advance, and it cannot be obtained by the accumulation of wealth alone, no matter how great. But the times are changing, and the indications are many that this civilisation has begun to pass from the age of pure materialism to a desire for the realities and truths of the universe. The general and rapidly increasing interest exhibited today for knowledge of superphysical truths, the growing number of those who are desiring information on existence before and after this life, the founding of methods to conquer disease by faith and spiritual means, the quest after the ancient teachings and wisdom of the East – all these are signs that people of the present time have glimpsed the reality of things. Thus, when we come to the problem of healing we can understand that this also will have to keep pace with the times and change its methods from those of gross materialism to those of a science founded upon the realities of Truth and governed by the same Divine laws which rule our very natures. Healing will pass from the domain of physical methods of treating the physical body to that of spiritual and mental healing, which, by bringing about harmony between the Soul and mind, will eradicate the very basic cause of disease, and then allow such physical means to be used as may be necessary to complete the cure of the body.

It seems quite possible that unless the medical profession realises these facts and advances with the spiritual growth of the people the art of healing may pass into the hands of religious orders or into those of the trueborn healers of men who exist in every generation, but who yet have lived more or less unobserved, prevented from following their natural calling by the attitude of the orthodox. So that the physician of the future will have two great aims. The first will be to assist the patient to a knowledge of himself and to point out to him the fundamental mistakes he may be making, the deficiencies in his character which he should remedy, and the defects in his nature which must be eradicated and replaced by the corresponding virtues. Such a physician will have to be a great student of the laws governing humanity and of human nature itself, so that he may recognise in all who come to him those elements which are causing a conflict between the Soul and the personality. He must be able to advise the sufferer how best to bring about the harmony required, what actions against Unity he must cease to perform and the necessary virtues he must develop to wipe out his defects. Each case will need a careful study, and it will only be those who have devoted much of their life to the knowledge of mankind and in whose heart burns the desire to help, who will be able to undertake successfully this glorious and divine work for humanity, to open the eyes of a sufferer and enlighten him on the reason of his being, and to inspire hope, comfort and faith which will enable him to conquer his malady.

The second duty of the physician will be to administer such remedies as will help the physical body to gain strength and assist the mind to become calm, widen its outlook and strive towards perfection, thus bringing peace and harmony to the whole personality. Such remedies there are in nature, placed there by the mercy of the Divine Creator for the healing and comfort of mankind. A few of these are known, and more are being sought at the present time by physicians in different parts of the world, especially in our Mother India, and there is no doubt that when such researches have become more developed we shall regain much of the knowledge which was known more than two thousand years ago, and the healer of the future will have at his disposal the wonderful and natural remedies which were divinely placed for man to relieve his sickness.

Thus the abolition of disease will depend upon humanity realising the truth of the unalterable laws of our Universe and adapting itself with humility and obedience to those laws, thus bringing peace between its Soul and itself, and gaining the real joy and happiness of life. And the part of the physician will be to assist any sufferer to a knowledge of such truth and to point out to him the means by which he can gain harmony, to inspire him with faith in his Divinity which can overcome all, and to administer such physical remedies as will help in the harmonising of the personality and the healing of the body.

# CHAPTER SEVEN

And now we come to the all-important problem, how can we help ourselves? How can we keep our mind and body in that state of harmony which will make it difficult or impossible for disease to attack us, for it is certain that the personality without conflict is immune from illness.

First let us consider the mind. We have already discussed at some length the necessity of seeking within ourselves those defects we possess which cause us to work against Unity and out of harmony with the dictates of the Soul, and of eliminating these faults by developing the opposing virtues. This can be done on the lines already indicated, and an honest self-examination will disclose to us the nature of our errors. Our spiritual advisers, true physicians and intimate friends should all be able to assist us to obtain a faithful picture of ourselves, but the perfect method of learning this is by calm thought and meditation, and by bringing ourselves to such an atmosphere of peace that our Souls are able to speak to us through our conscience and intuition, and to guide us according to their wishes. If we can only set aside a short time every day, quite alone and in as quiet a place as possible, free from interruption, and merely sit or lie quietly, either keeping the mind a blank or calmly thinking of one's work in life, it will be found after a time that we get great help at such moments and, as it were, flashes of knowledge and guidance are given to us. We find that the questions of the difficult problems of life are unmistakably answered, and we become able to choose with confidence the right course. Throughout such times we should keep an earnest desire in the heart to serve humanity and work according to the dictates of our Soul.

Be it remembered that when the fault is found the remedy lies not in a battle against this and not in a use of will power and energy to suppress a wrong, but in a steady development of the opposite virtue, thus automatically washing from our natures all trace of the offender. This is the true and natural method of advancement and of the conquest of wrong, vastly easier and more effective than fighting a particular defect. To struggle against a fault increases its power, keeps our attention riveted on its presence, and brings us a battle indeed, and the most success we can then expect is conquest by suppression, which is far from satisfactory, as the enemy is still with us and may in a weak moment show itself afresh. To forget the failing and consciously to strive to develop the virtue which would make the former impossible, this is true victory.

For example, should there be cruelty in our nature, we can continually say, "I will not be cruel", and so prevent ourselves erring in that direction; but the success of this depends on the strength of the mind, and should it weaken we might for the moment forget our good resolve. But should we, on the other hand, develop real sympathy towards our fellow-men, this quality will once and for all make cruelty impossible, for we should shun the very act with horror because of our fellow-feeling. About this there is no suppression, no hidden enemy to come forward at moments when we are off our guard, because our sympathy will have completely eradicated from our nature the possibility of any act which could hurt another.

As we have previously seen, the nature of our physical maladies will materially help in pointing out to us the mental disharmony which is the basic cause of their origin; and another great factor of success is that we must have a zest for life and look upon existence not merely as a duty to be borne with as much patience as possible, developing a real joy in the adventure of our journey through this world.

Perhaps one of the greatest tragedies of materialism is the development of boredom and the loss of real inner happiness; it teaches people to seek contentment and compensation for troubles in earthly enjoyments and pleasures, and these can never bring anything but temporary oblivion of our difficulties. Once we begin to seek compensation for our trials at the hands of the paid jester we start a vicious circle. Amusement, entertainment and frivolity are good for us all, but not when we persistently depend upon these to alleviate our troubles. Worldly amusements of every kind have to be steadily increased in their intensity to keep their hold, and the thrill of yesterday becomes the bore of to-morrow. So we go on seeking other and greater excitements until we become satiated and can no longer obtain relief in that direction. In some form or another reliance on worldly entertainment makes Fausts of us all, and though perhaps we may not fully realise it in our conscious self, life becomes for us little more than a patient duty and all its true zest and joy, such as should be the heritage of every child and be maintained until our latest hours, departs from us. The extreme stage is reached today in the scientific efforts being evolved to obtain rejuvenation, prolongation of natural life and increase of sensual pleasures by means of devilish practices.

The state of boredom is responsible for the admittance into ourselves of much more disease than would be generally realised, and as it tends today to occur early in life, so the maladies associated with it tend to appear at a younger age. Such a conditioncannot occur if we acknowledge the truth of our Divinity, our mission in the world, and thereby possess the joy of gaining experience and helping others. The antidote for boredom is to take an active and lively interest in all around us, to study life throughout the whole day, to learn and learn and learn from our fellow-men and from the occurrences in life the Truth that lies behind all things, to lose ourselves in the art of gaining knowledge and experience, and to watch for opportunities when we may use such to the advantage of a fellow-traveller. Thus every moment of our work and play will bring with it a zeal for learning, a desire to experience real things, real adventures and deeds worth while, and as we develop this faculty we shall find that we are regaining the power of obtaining joy from the smallest incidents, and occurrences we have previously regarded as commonplace and of dull monotony will become the opportunity for research and adventure. It is in the simple things of life – the simple things because they are nearer the great Truth– that real pleasure is to be found.

Resignation, which makes one become merely an unobservant passenger on the journey of life, opens the door to untold adverse influences which would never have an opportunity of gaining admittance as long as our daily existence brought with it the spirit and joy of adventure. Whatever may be our station, whether a worker in the city with its teeming myriads or a lonely shepherd on the hills, let us strive to turn monotony into interest, dull duty into a joyous opportunity for experience, and daily life into an intense study of humanity and the great fundamental laws of the Universe. In every place there is ample opportunity to observe the laws of Creation, either in the mountains or valleys or amongst our brother men. First let us turn life into an adventure of absorbing interest, when boredom will be no longer possible, and from the knowledge thus gained seek to harmonise our mind with our Soul and with the great Unity of God's Creation.

Another fundamental help to us is to put away all fear. Fear in reality holds no place in the natural human kingdom, since the Divinity within us, which is ourself, is unconquerable and immortal, and if we could but realise it we, as Children of God, have nothing of which to be afraid. In materialistic ages fear naturally increases in earthly possessions (whether they be of the body itself or external riches), for if such things be our world, since they are so transient, so difficult to obtain and so impossible to hold save for a brief spell, they arouse in us the utmost anxiety lest we miss an opportunity of grasping them while we may, and we must of necessity live in a constant state of fear, conscious or subconscious, because in our inner self we know that such possessions may at any moment be snatched from us and that at the most we can only hold them for a brief life.

In this age the fear of disease has developed until it has become a great power for harm, because it opens the door to those things we dread and makes it easier for their admission. Such fear is really self-interest, for when we are earnestly absorbed in the welfare of others there is no time to be apprehensive of personal maladies. Fear at the present time is playing a great part in intensifying disease, and modern science has increased the reign of terror by spreading abroad to the general public its discoveries, which as yet are but half-truths. The knowledge of bacteria and the various germs associated with disease has played havoc in the minds of tens of thousands of people, and by the dread aroused in them has in itself rendered them more susceptible of attack. While lower forms of life, such as bacteria, may play a part in or be associated with physical disease, they constitute by no means the whole truth of the problem, as can be demonstrated scientifically or by everyday occurrences. There is a factor which science is unable to explain on physical grounds, and that is why some people become affected by disease whilst others escape, although both classes may be open to the same possibility of infection. Materialism forgets that there is a factor above the physical plane which in the ordinary course of life protects or renders susceptible any particular individual with regard to disease, of whatever nature it may be. Fear, by its depressing effect on our mentality, thus causing disharmony in our physical and magnetic bodies, paves the way for invasion, and if bacteria and such physical means were the sure and only cause of disease, then indeed there might be but little encouragement not to be afraid. But when we realise that in the worst epidemics only a proportion of those exposed to infection are attacked and that, as we have already seen, the real cause of disease lies in our own personality and is within our control, then have we reason to go about without dread and fearless, knowing that the remedy lies with ourselves. We can put all fear of physical means alone as a cause of disease out of our minds, knowing that such anxiety merely renders as susceptible, and that if we are endeavouring to bring harmony into our personality we need anticipate illness no more than we dread being struck by lightning or hit by a fragment of a falling meteor.

Now let us consider the physical body. It must never be forgotten that this is but the earthly habitation of the Soul, in which we dwell only for a short time in order that we may be able to contact the world for the purpose of gaining experience and knowledge. Without too much identifying ourselves with our bodies we should treat them with respect and care, so that they may be healthy and last the longer to do our work. Never for one moment should we become engrossed or over-anxious about them, but learn to be as little conscious of their existence as possible, using them as a vehicle of our Soul and mind and as servants to do our will. External and internal cleanliness are of great importance. For the former we of the West use our water too hot; this opens the skin and allows the admission of dirt. Moreover, the excessive use of soap renders the surface sticky. Cool or tepid water, either running as a shower bath or changed more than once is nearer the natural method and keeps the body healthier; only such an amount of soap as is necessary to remove obvious dirt should be used, and this should afterwards be well washed off in fresh water.

Internal cleanliness depends on diet, and we should choose everything that is clean and wholesome and as fresh as possible, chiefly natural fruits, vegetables and nuts. Animal flesh should certainly be avoided; first, because it gives rise to much physical poison in the body; secondly, because it stimulates an abnormal and excessive appetite; and thirdly, because it necessitates cruelty to the animal world. Plenty of fluid should be taken to cleanse the body, such as water and natural wines and products made direct from Nature's storehouse, avoiding the more

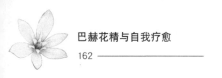
artificial beverages of distillation.

Sleep should not be excessive, as many of us have more control over ourselves whilst awake than when asleep. The old saying, "Time to turn over, time to turn out", is an excellent guide as to when to rise.

Clothing should be as light in weight as is compatible with warmth; it should allow air to reach the body, and sunshine and fresh air should be permitted to contact the skin on all possible occasions. Water and sun bathing are great donors of health and vitality.

In all things cheerfulness should be encouraged, and we should refuse to be oppressed by doubt and depression, but remember that such are not of ourselves, for our Souls know only joy and happiness.

# CHAPTER EIGHT

Thus we see that our conquest of disease will mainly depend on the following: Firstly, the realisation of the Divinity within our nature and our consequent power to overcome all that is wrong: secondly, the knowledge that the basic cause of disease is due to disharmony between the personality and the Soul; thirdly, our willingness and ability to discover the fault which is causing such a conflict; and fourthly, the removal of any such fault by developing the opposing virtue.

The duty of the healing art will be to assist us to the necessary knowledge and means by which we may overcome our maladies, and in addition to this to administer such remedies as will strengthen our mental and physical bodies and give us greater opportunities of victory. Then shall we indeed be capable of attacking disease at its very base with real hope of success. The medical school of the future will not particularly interest itself in the ultimate results and products of disease, nor will it pay so much attention to actual physical lesions, or administer drugs and chemicals merely for the sake of palliating our symptoms, but knowing the true cause of sickness and aware that the obvious physical results are merely secondary, it will concentrate its efforts upon bringing about that harmony between body, mind and soul which results in the relief and cure of disease. And in such cases as are undertaken early enough the correction of the mind will avert the imminent illness.

Amongst the types of remedies that will be used will be those obtained from the most beautiful plants and herbs to be found in the pharmacy of Nature, such as have been divinely enriched with healing powers for the mind and body of man.

For our own part we must practise peace, harmony, individuality and firmness of purpose and increasingly develop the knowledge that in essence we are of Divine origin, children of the Creator, and thus have within us, if we will but develop it, as in time we ultimately surely must, the power to attain perfection. And this reality must increase within us until it becomes the most outstanding feature of our existence. We must steadfastly practise peace, imagining our minds as a lake ever to be kept calm, without waves, or even ripples, to disturb its tranquillity, and gradually develop this state of peace until no event of life, no circumstance, no other personality is able under any condition to ruffle the surface of that lake or raise within us any feelings of irritability, depression or doubt. It will materially help to set apart a short time each day to think quietly of the beauty of peace and the benefits of calmness, and to realise that it is neither by worrying nor hurrying that we accomplish most, but by calm, quiet thought and action become more efficient in all we undertake. To harmonise our conduct in this life in accordance with the wishes of our own Soul, and to remain in such a state of peace that the trials and disturbances of the world leave us unruffled, is a great attainment indeed and brings to us that Peace which passeth understanding; and though at first it may seem to be beyond our dreams, it is in reality, with patience and perseverance, within the reach of us all.

We are not all asked to be saints or martyrs or men of renown; to most of us less conspicuous offices are allotted. But we are all expected to understand the joy and adventures of life and to fulfil with cheerfulness the particular piece of work which has been ordained for us by our Divinity.

For those who are sick, peace of mind and harmony

with the Soul is the greatest aid to recovery. The medicine and nursing of the future will pay much more attention to the development of this within the patient than we do to-day when, unable to judge the progress of a case except by materialistic scientific means, we think more of the frequent taking of temperature and a number of attentions which interrupt, rather than promote, that quiet rest and relaxation of body and mind which are so essential to recovery. There is no doubt that at the very onset of, at any rate, minor ailments, if we could but get a few hours' complete relaxation and in harmony with our Higher Self the illness would be aborted. At such moments we need to bring down into ourselves but a fraction of that calm, as symbolised by the entry of Christ into the boat during the storm on the lake of Galilee, when He ordered "Peace, be still".

Our outlook on life depends on the nearness of the personality to the Soul. The closer the union the greater the harmony and peace, and the more clearly will shine the light of Truth and the radiant happiness which is of the higher realms; these will hold us steady and undismayed by the difficulties and terrors of the world, since they have their foundations on the Eternal Truth of Good. The knowledge of Truth also gives to us the certainty that, however tragic some of the events of the world may appear to be, they form but a temporary stage in the evolution of man; and that even disease is in itself beneficent and works under the operation of certain laws designed to produce ultimate good and exerting a continual pressure towards perfection. Those who have this knowledge are unable to be touched or depressed or dismayed by those events which are such a burden to others, and all uncertainty, fear and despair go for ever. If we can but keep in constant communion with our own Soul, our Heavenly Father, then indeed is the world a place of joy, nor can any adverse influence be exerted upon us.

We are not permitted to see the magnitude of our own Divinity, or to realise the mightiness of our Destiny and the glorious future which lies before us; for, if we were, life would be no trial and would involve no effort, no test of merit. Our virtue lies in being oblivious for the most part to those great things, and yet having faith and courage to live well and master the difficulties of this earth. We can, however, by communion with our Higher Self, keep that harmony which enables us to overcome all worldly opposition and make our journey along the straight path to fulfil our destiny, undeterred by the influences which would lead us astray.

Next must we develop individuality and free ourselves from all worldly influences, so that obeying only the dictates of our own Soul and unmoved by circumstances or other people we become our own masters, steering our bark over the rough seas of life without ever quitting the helm of rectitude, or at any time leaving the steering of our vessel to the hands of another. We must gain our freedom absolutely and completely, so that all we do, our every action – nay, even our every thought – derives its origin in ourselves, thus enabling us to live and give freely of our own accord, and of our own accord alone.

Our greatest difficulty in this direction may lie with those nearest to us in this age when the fear of convention and false standards of duty are so appallingly developed. But we must increase our courage, which with so many of us is sufficient to face the apparently big things of life, but which yet fails at the more intimate trials. We must be able with impersonality to determine right and wrong and to act fearlessly in the presence of relative or friend. What a vast number of us are heroes in the outer world, but cowards at home! Though subtle indeed may be the means used to prevent us from fulfilling our Destiny, the pretence of love and affection, or a false sense of duty, methods to enslave us and keep us prisoners to the wishes and desires of others, yet must all such be ruthlessly put aside. The voice of our own Soul, and that voice alone, must be heeded as regards our duty if we are not to be hampered by those around us. Individuality must be developed to the utmost, and we must learn to walk through life relying on none but our own Soul for guidance and help, to take our freedom with both hands and plunge into the world to gain every particle of knowledge and experience which may be possible.

At the same time we must be on our guard to allow to everyone their freedom also, to expect nothing from others, but, on the contrary, to be ever ready to lend a helping hand to lift them upwards in times of their need and difficulty. Thus every personality we meet in life, whether mother, husband, child, stranger or friend, becomes a fellow-traveller, and any one of them may be greater or smaller than ourselves as regards spiritual development; but all of us are members of a common brotherhood and part of a great community making the same journey and with the same glorious end in view.

We must be steadfast in the determination to win, resolute

in the will to gain the mountain summit; let us not give a moment's regret to the slips by the way. No great ascent was ever made without faults and falls, and they must be regarded as experiences which will help us to stumble less in the future. No thoughts of past errors must ever depress us; they are over and finished, and the knowledge thus gained will help to avoid a repetition of them. Steadily must we press forwards and onwards, never regretting and never looking back, for the past of even one hour ago is behind us, and the glorious future with its blazing light ever before us. All fear must be cast out; it should never exist in the human mind, and is only possible when we lose sight of our Divinity. It is foreign to us because as Sons of the Creator, Sparks of the Divine Life, we are invincible, indestructible and unconquerable. Disease is apparently cruel because it is the penalty of wrong thought and wrong action, which must result in cruelty to others. Hence the necessity of developing the love and brotherhood side of our natures to the utmost, since this will make cruelty in the future an impossibility.

The development of Love brings us to the realisation of Unity, of the truth that one and all of us are of the One Great

Creation.

The cause of all our troubles is self and separateness, and this vanishes as soon as Love and the knowledge of the great Unity become part of our natures. The Universe is God rendered objective; at its birth it is God reborn; at its close it is God more highly evolved. So with man; his body is himself externalised, an objective manifestation of his internal nature; he is the expression of himself, the materialisation of the qualities of his consciousness.

In our Western civilisation we have the glorious example, the great standard of perfection and the teachings of the Christ to guide us. He acts for us as Mediator between our personality and our Soul. His mission on earth was to teach us how to obtain harmony and communion with our Higher Self, with Our Father which is in Heaven, and thereby to obtain perfection in accordance with the Will of the Great Creator of all.

Thus also taught the Lord Buddha and other great Masters who have come down from time to time upon the earth to point out to men the way to attain perfection. There is no halfway path for humanity. The Truth must be acknowledged, and man must unite himself with the infinite scheme of Love of his Creator.

And so come out, my brothers and sisters, into the glorious sunshine of the knowledge of your Divinity, and earnestly and steadfastly set to work to join in the Grand Design of being happy and communicating happiness, uniting with that great band of the White Brotherhood[1] whose whole existence is to obey the wish of their God, and whose great joy is in the service of their younger brother men.

---

[1] See the Foreword

附录3

# 第二部英文版

## The Twelve Healers and
## Other Remedies

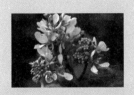

Edward Bach

# The Twelve Healers and Other Remedies

*The definitive edition*

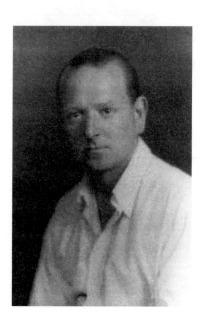

*This work of healing has been done and published and given freely so that people like yourselves can help yourselves, either in illness or to keep well and strong.*

- Edward Bach, speaking on his 50th birthday

24th September 1936

# EDITORS' INTRODUCTION

The roots of *The Twelve Healers and Other Remedies* lie in the February 1930 issue of the journal *Homoeopathic World*. Here, under the title "Some New Remedies and New Uses", the doctor-turned-homoeopath Edward Bach published an account of five plant-based remedies, of which three – Impatiens, Mimulus and Clematis – would be the starting point of the Bach flower remedy system. These remedies were homoeopathic preparations, prepared using trituration and succussion. Flower remedies as we now know them began later that same year, with the discovery of the sun method of preparation.

By 1932 the number of remedies had grown to twelve, and Bach included an account of them in a booklet called *Free Thyself*. In the following spring, 1933, he was already looking for more remedies, but found time to write and publish further, including two articles, "Twelve Great Remedies" and "Twelve Healers", the latter printed in Epsom, and a booklet, *The Twelve*

*Healers*, printed in Marlow. Many years later, Nora Weeks recalled how this last manuscript

...was printed locally in pamphlet form, and he [Bach] decided to sell it at twopence a copy in order that all could afford to buy it and benefit from the herbal remedies. He hoped in this way to cover the cost of printing the pamphlet, for, as usual, he had little money to spare; but he never did: he would send copies to all who asked for them, always forgetting to ask for two pennies in exchange.[①]

In August 1933 Bach wrote to The CW Daniel Company, who had published his book *Heal Thyself* a couple of years before. He sent them a copy of his *The Twelve Healers* pamphlet, and some additional typewritten material headed "The Four Helpers", which introduced new remedies found that year. Daniels published *The Twelve Healers* and Four Helpers that autumn; and a year later, in July 1934, brought out a second

————————————

[①]　Nora Weeks, *The Medical Discoveries of Edward Bach*, chapter XVI.

edition that included a further three remedies: *The Twelve Healers and Seven Helpers.*

By the autumn of 1935 Bach had discovered a further nineteen remedies, along with the boiling method of preparation. With a total of 38 remedies he announced that the system was complete. He wrote to The CW Daniel Company and asked them, as a stopgap, to print a two-page leaflet with brief information on the new remedies and insert it into the remaining stock of *The Twelve Healers and Seven Helpers*. Soon he was at work on a new, final version of the book.

This last edition saw a complete change in the presentation of the remedies. Starting with the first CW Daniel edition, Bach had drawn a distinction between *healers* (twelve fundamental remedies), and *helpers* (seven remedies for long-term states, used when the choice of healer wasn't clear). Now that he had to incorporate another nineteen remedies into the system, he theorised that each new remedy might correspond to one of the healers or helpers.

He laboured on this design for some time – but it was never completed. Perhaps it got in the way of that perfect simplicity which felt so right to him. Perhaps some remedies didn't fall naturally into place. Almost certainly, he doubted whether the arrangement was of any practical use: the "thirty-eight different states... simply described" were enough "to find that state or a mixture of states which are present, and so to be able to give the required remedies." [1] Did it really matter whether people ended up with healers or helpers, or neither, or both?

In the end, Bach removed the healers/helpers distinction entirely, and instead classified the 38 remedies under seven general headings. He was so thorough in his revision that his publishers were concerned at the effect of such a change on the book's readers. They wrote back to the author:

> We note that you retain the title, The Twelve Healers, but the book in its present form does not indicate what are the Twelve Healers. We suggest that the Twelve Healers should be indicated by an asterisk and that a note of this fact should be made in the Introduction. [2]

---

[1]　From Bach's Introduction to *The Twelve Healers and Other Remedies*; see page 13.

[2]　Letter from The CW Daniel Co Ltd to Edward Bach, 27th July 1936.

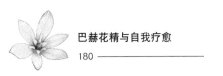
Bach ignored the request to highlight the first twelve, but did add a couple of sentences to the end of the Introduction to account for the title. At the proof stage, the publishers went ahead and inserted asterisks themselves, and added their own final sentence:

We have [...] taken the liberty of adding to your additional note to Introduction the following: "The original twelve are indicated by asterisks." We have added the asterisks to the names in the Remedies Section *[sic]* and in the list of names. [1]

The finished book, *The Twelve Healers and Other Remedies*, was published on Bach's 50th birthday, September 24th 1936. In accordance with the author's instructions, the publishers withdrew and destroyed remaining stocks of the previous edition. As Nora Weeks recalled,

---

[1] Letter from The CW Daniel Co Ltd to Edward Bach, dated 31st July 1936.

It had always been his custom to destroy any notes made during the course of his researches directly he had reached the final conclusion and published the result. He felt in this way there would be no conflicting accounts to puzzle the learner; his aim being to make the healing of disease a simple matter, and so remove the fear present in the minds of most at the thought of illness. [1]

The 1936 edition was the last prepared in Dr Bach's lifetime. But only weeks after its publication, he was writing of the need to adapt it, to do more to defend the simplicity of the completed system. "When the next edition of *The Twelve Healers* becomes necessary," he wrote to his friend Victor Bullen, "we must have a longer introduction, firmly upholding the harmlessness, the simplicity and the miraculous healing powers of the Remedies." [2]

Bach dictated this longer introduction to his assistant Nora Weeks on the 30th of October 1936. It was one of the last acts

---

[1]　Nora Weeks, *The Medical Discoveries of Edward Bach*, chapter XX.

[2]　Letter to Victor Bullen dated 26th October 1936.

of his life. A month later, on November 27th, he died in his sleep.

As she had promised to do, Nora Weeks sent the new material to The CW Daniel Company early in December 1936. It was the only significant change made when the 1941 edition was printed, so that this text, all in Dr Bach's own words [1], can be considered the definitive version of the book.

*The Twelve Healers and Other Remedies* has been in print ever since. It has been translated into most major languages – not always successfully – and has gone through countless editions. Over the years, the original remedy descriptions remained sacrosanct [2] . But other parts of the text were open to editing and updating. Following Bach's own lead, the custodians of the Bach Centre always treated *The Twelve Healers* as a living text whose job was to present and preserve the simplicity of the system.

The world has changed, though, and it no longer seems

---

[1]  Apart from minor changes to one section made by Nora Weeks for the 1941 edition: see the footnote on page 34.

[2]  An exception was the removal of one sentence from Bach's description of Rock Rose – see the footnote in the main text.

so important to keep *The Twelve Healers* updated in quite the same way. We have other ways to present detailed information about dosage and working with animals and so on: web sites; social networks; training courses; and specialist books on everything from selecting remedies for horses to making your own.

The challenge today is more about honouring Edward Bach's original work, and his wishes for its future. He would have been disappointed that pre-1936 editions have been republished and used to reinterpret and complicate the finished system. We feel the time is right, then, to put the emphasis back onto the definitive 1941 edition, with not a word changed, and with notes to guide the reader below the surface of the text.

At the same time we are working with Bach Foundation Registered Practitioners around the world to produce new translations of this seminal work into as many languages as possible. Many of the existing translations contain grave errors, and the preparation of definitive foreign-language editions is long overdue.

The autumn of 2011, which sees the 75<sup>th</sup> anniversary of

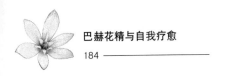

Dr Bach's death and the 125<sup>th</sup> anniversary of his birth, seems a fitting time to offer this gift.

Judy Ramsell Howard

Stefan Ball

# INTRODUCTION

This system of treatment is the most perfect which has been given to mankind within living memory. [①] It has the power to cure disease; and, in its simplicity, it may be used in the household.

It is its simplicity, combined with its all-healing effects, that is so wonderful.

No science, no knowledge is necessary, apart from the simple methods described herein; and they who will obtain the greatest benefit from this God-sent Gift will be those who keep it pure as it is; free from science, free from theories, for everything in Nature is simple.

This system of healing, which has been Divinely revealed unto us, shows that it is our fears, our cares, our anxieties and

———————————

[①]　The first seven paragraphs of the Introduction were dictated by Bach after the 1936 edition was published. See the Editors' Introduction for more information.

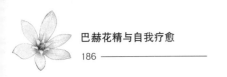

such like that open the path to the invasion of illness. Thus by treating our fears, our cares, our worries and so on, we not only free ourselves from our illness, but the Herbs given unto us by the Grace of the Creator of all, in addition take away our fears and worries, and leave us happier and better in ourselves.

As the Herbs heal our fears, our anxieties, our worries, our faults and our failings, it is these we must seek, and then the disease, no matter what it is, will leave us.

There is little more to say, for the understanding mind will know all this, and may there be sufficient of those with understanding minds, unhampered by the trend of science, to use these Gifts of God for the relief and the blessing of those around them.

Thus, behind all disease lie our fears, our anxieties, our greed, our likes and dislikes. Let us seek these out and heal them, and with the healing of them will go the disease from which we suffer.

From time immemorial it has been known that Providential Means has placed in Nature the prevention and cure of disease, by means of divinely enriched herbs and plants and trees. [①] The remedies of Nature given in this book have proved that they are blest above others in their work of mercy; and that they have been given the power to heal all types of illness and suffering.

In treating cases with these remedies no notice is taken of the nature of the disease. The individual is treated, and as he becomes well the disease goes, having been cast off by the increase of health.

All know that the same disease may have different effects on different people; it is the effects that need treatment, because they guide to the real cause.

The mind being the most delicate and sensitive part of the body, shows the onset and the course of disease much more definitely than the body, so that the outlook of mind is chosen as the guide as to which remedy or remedies are necessary.

In illness there is a change of mood from that in ordinary life, and those who are observant can notice this change often before, and sometimes long before, the disease appears, and by

---

[①]　This sentence marks the start of the shorter introduction that appeared in the 1936 edition.

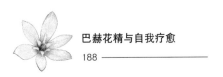

treatment can prevent the malady ever appearing. When illness has been present for some time, again the mood of the sufferer will guide to the correct remedy.

Take no notice of the disease, think only of the outlook on life of the one in distress.

Thirty-eight different states are simply described: and there should be no difficulty either for oneself, or for another, to find that state or a mixture of states which are present, and so to be able to give the required remedies to effect a cure.

The title, [①] *The Twelve Healers*, has been retained for this book, as it is familiar to many readers.

The relief of suffering was so certain and beneficial, even when there were only twelve remedies, that it was deemed necessary to bring these before the attention of the public at the time, without waiting for the discovery of the remaining twenty-six, which complete the series. The original twelve are indicated by asterisks.

---

[①]    This and the subsequent paragraph were added to the typescript of the 1936 edition at the proof stage. See the Editors' Introduction.

# THE REMEDIES

## And the reasons given for each [1]

---

[1] Cf. the 1936 edition, which has "The Remedies and the reasons for giving each" . The change in wording was probably a printer's error.

# THE 38 REMEDIES
# are placed under the following
# 7 HEADINGS[1]

1. FOR FEAR

2. FOR UNCERTAINTY

3. FOR INSUFFICIENT INTEREST IN PRESENT CIRCUMSTANCES

4. FOR LONELINESS

5. FOR THOSE OVER-SENSITIVE TO INFLUENCES AND IDEAS

6. FOR DESPONDENCY OR DESPAIR

7. FOR OVER-CARE[2]  FOR WELFARE OF OTHERS

---

[1]  The group names are based on the general emotional characteristics Bach identified for each of the seven Bach nosodes. The Bach nosodes were a set of homoeopathic remedies made from bacteria, which Bach worked on between 1919 and 1928. See Nora Weeks, *The Medical Discoveries of Edward Bach*, chapters V and VI.

[2]  The 1941 edition capitalises this as "Over-Care"; for the current edition we have amended this to follow the pattern set two lines before by "Over-sensitive".

# FOR THOSE WHO HAVE FEAR

## *ROCK ROSE

The rescue remedy. [①] The remedy of emergency for cases where there even appears no hope. In accident or sudden illness, or when the patient is very frightened or terrified, or if the condition is serious enough to cause great fear to those around. If the patient is not conscious the lips may be moistened with the remedy. Other remedies in addition may also be required, as, for example, if there is unconsciousness, which is a deep, sleepy state, Clematis; if there is torture, Agrimony, and so on.

## *MIMULUS

Fear of worldly things, illness, pain, accidents, poverty, of

————————————

[①]　This first sentence was omitted from most later editions of the book. Dr. Bach combined five remedies and called it "rescue remedy", and some readers were confused that the same name was also used to describe Rock Rose.

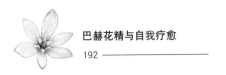
dark, of being alone, of misfortune. The fears of everyday life. These people quietly and secretly bear their dread, they do not freely speak of it to others.

## CHERRY PLUM

Fear of the mind being over-strained, of reason giving way, of doing fearful and dreaded things, not wished and known wrong, yet there comes the thought and impulse to do them.

## ASPEN

Vague unknown fears, for which there can be given no explanation, no reason.

Yet the patient may be terrified of something terrible going to happen, he knows not what.

These vague unexplainable fears may haunt by night or day.

Sufferers often are afraid to tell their trouble to others.

## RED CHESTNUT

For those who find it difficult not to be anxious for other people.

Often they have ceased to worry about themselves, but for those of whom they are fond they may suffer much, frequently anticipating that some unfortunate thing may happen to them.

## FOR THOSE WHO SUFFER UNCERTAINTY

### *CERATO

Those who have not sufficient confidence in themselves to make their own decisions.

They constantly seek advice from others, and are often misguided.

### *SCLERANTHUS

Those who suffer much from being unable to decide between two things, first one seeming right then the other.

They are usually quiet people, and bear their difficulty alone, as they are not inclined to discuss it with others.

### *GENTIAN

Those who are easily discouraged. They may be

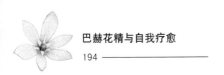

progressing well in illness or in the affairs of their daily life, but any small delay or hindrance to progress causes doubt and soon disheartens them.

## GORSE

Very great hopelessness, they have given up belief that more can be done for them.

Under persuasion or to please others they may try different treatments, at the same time assuring those around that there is so little hope of relief.

## HORNBEAM

For those who feel that they have not sufficient strength, mentally or physically, to carry the burden of life placed upon them; the affairs of every day seem too much for them to accomplish, though they generally succeed in fulfilling their task.

For those who believe that some part, of mind or body, needs to be strengthened before they can easily fulfil their work.

## WILD OAT

Those who have ambitions to do something of prominence

in life, who wish to have much experience, and to enjoy all that which is possible for them, to take life to the full.

Their difficulty is to determine what occupation to follow; as although their ambitions are strong, they have no calling which appeals to them above all others.

This may cause delay and dissatisfaction.

## NOT SUFFICIENT INTEREST IN PRESENT CIRCUMSTANCES

### *CLEMATIS

Those who are dreamy, drowsy, not fully awake, no great interest in life. Quiet people, not really happy in their present circumstances, living more in the future than in the present; living in hopes of happier times, when their ideals may come true. In illness some make little or no effort to get well, and in certain cases may even look forward to death, in the hope of better times; or maybe, meeting again some beloved one whom they have lost.

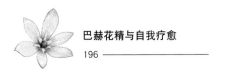
## HONEYSUCKLE

Those who live much in the past, perhaps a time of great happiness, or memories of a lost friend, or ambitions which have not come true. They do not expect further happiness such as they have had.

## WILD ROSE

Those who without apparently sufficient reason become resigned to all that happens, and just glide through life, take it as it is, without any effort to improve things and find some joy. They have surrendered to the struggle of life without complaint.

## OLIVE

Those who have suffered much mentally or physically and are so exhausted and weary that they feel they have no more strength to make any effort. Daily life is hard work for them, without pleasure.

## WHITE CHESTNUT

For those who cannot prevent thoughts, ideas, arguments

which they do not desire from entering their minds. Usually at such times when the interest of the moment is not strong enough to keep the mind full.

Thoughts which worry and will remain, or if for a time thrown out, will return. They seem to circle round and round and cause mental torture.

The presence of such unpleasant thoughts drives out peace and interferes with being able to think only of the work or pleasure of the day.

## MUSTARD

Those who are liable to times of gloom, or even despair, as though a cold dark cloud overshadowed them and hid the light and the joy of life. It may not be possible to give any reason or explanation for such attacks.

Under these conditions it is almost impossible to appear happy or cheerful.

## CHESTNUT BUD

For those who do not take full advantage of observation and experience, and who take a longer time than others to learn

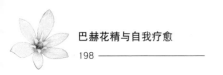

the lessons of daily life.

Whereas one experience would be enough for some, such people find it necessary to have more, sometimes several, before the lesson is learnt.

Therefore, to their regret, they find themselves having to make the same error on different occasions when once would have been enough, or observation of others could have spared them even that one fault.

## LONELINESS

### *WATER VIOLET

For those who in health or illness like to be alone. Very quiet people, who move about without noise, speak little, and then gently. Very independent, capable and self-reliant. Almost free of the opinions of others. They are aloof, leave people alone and go their own way. Often clever and talented. Their peace and calmness is a blessing to those around them.

## *IMPATIENS

Those who are quick in thought and action and who wish all things to be done without hesitation or delay. When ill they are anxious for a hasty recovery.

They find it very difficult to be patient with people who are slow, as they consider it wrong and a waste of time, and they will endeavour to make such people quicker in all ways.

They often prefer to work and think alone, so that they can do everything at their own speed.

## HEATHER

Those who are always seeking the companionship of anyone who may be available, as they find it necessary to discuss their own affairs with others, no matter whom it may be. They are very unhappy if they have to be alone for any length of time.

# OVER-SENSITIVE TO INFLUENCES AND IDEAS

## *AGRIMONY

The jovial, cheerful, humorous people who love peace and

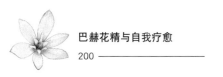

are distressed by argument or quarrel, to avoid which they will agree to give up much.

Though generally they have troubles and are tormented and restless and worried in mind or in body, they hide their cares behind their humour and jesting and are considered very good friends to know. They often take alcohol or drugs in excess, to stimulate themselves and help themselves bear their trials with cheerfulness.

### *CENTAURY

Kind, quiet, gentle people who are over-anxious to serve others. They overtax their strength in their endeavours.

Their wish so grows upon them that they become more servants than willing helpers. Their good nature leads them to do more than their own share of work, and in so doing they may neglect their own particular mission in life.

### WALNUT

For those who have definite ideals and ambitions in life and are fulfilling them, but on rare occasions are tempted to be led away from their own ideas, aims and work by the enthusiasm, convictions or strong opinions of others.

The remedy gives constancy and protection from outside influences.

### HOLLY

For those who sometimes are attacked by thoughts of such kind as jealousy, envy, revenge, suspicion.

For the different forms of vexation.

Within themselves they may suffer much, often when there is no real cause for their unhappiness.

## FOR DESPONDENCY OR DESPAIR

### LARCH

For those who do not consider themselves as good or capable as those around them, who expect failure, who feel that they will never be a success, and so do not venture or make a strong enough attempt to succeed.

### PINE

For those who blame themselves. Even when successful

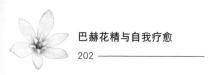

they think that①  they could have done better, and are never content with their efforts or the results. They are hard-working and suffer much from the faults they attach to themselves.

Sometimes if there is any mistake it is due to another, but they will claim responsibility even for that.

## ELM

Those who are doing good work, are following the calling of their life and who hope to do something of importance, and this often for the benefit of humanity.

At times there may be periods of depression when they feel that the task they have undertaken is too difficult, and not within the power of a human being.

## SWEET CHESTNUT

For those moments which happen to some people when the anguish is so great as to seem to be unbearable.

When the mind or body feels as if it had borne to the uttermost limit of its endurance, and that now it must give way.

---

① The word "that" is omitted from most later editions.

When it seems there is nothing but destruction and annihilation left to face.

## STAR OF BETHLEHEM

For those in great distress under conditions which for a time produce great unhappiness.

The shock of serious news, the loss of some one[①] dear, the fright following an accident, and such like.

For those who for a time refuse to be consoled[②] this remedy brings comfort.

## WILLOW

For those who have suffered adversity or misfortune and find these difficult to accept, without complaint or resentment, as they judge life much by the success which it brings.

They feel that they have not deserved so great a trial, that it was unjust, and they become embittered.

---

[①]　In subsequent editions "some one" is usually written as "someone". We have preferred "some one" as it matches Bach's usage in the description for Clematis, where he writes of "some beloved one".

[②]　Most later editions insert a comma after "consoled".

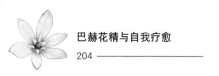
They often take less interest and less activity[1] in those things of life which they had previously enjoyed.

## OAK

For those who are struggling and fighting strongly to get well, or in connection with the affairs of their daily life. They will go on trying one thing after another, though their case may seem hopeless.

They will fight on. They are discontented with themselves if illness interferes with their duties or helping others.

They are brave people, fighting against great difficulties, without loss of hope or effort.

## CRAB APPLE

This is the remedy of cleansing.

For those who feel as if they had something not quite clean about themselves.

Often it is something of apparently little importance:

---

[1] Most later editions give this sentence as "They often take less interest and are less active..."

in others there may be more serious disease which is almost disregarded compared to the one thing on which they concentrate.

In both types they are anxious to be free from the one particular thing which is greatest in their minds and which seems so essential to them that it should be cured.

They become despondent if treatment fails.

Being a cleanser, this remedy purifies wounds if the patient has reason to believe that some poison has entered which must be drawn out.

## OVER-CARE FOR WELFARE OF OTHERS

### *CHICORY

Those who are very mindful of the needs of others; they tend to be over-full of care for children, relatives, friends, always finding something that should be put right. They are continually correcting what they consider wrong, and enjoy doing so. They desire that those for whom they care should be near them.

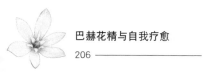
## *VERVAIN

Those with fixed principles and ideas, which they are confident are right, and which they very rarely change.

They have a great wish to convert all around them to their own views of life.

They are strong of will and have much courage when they are convinced of those things that they wish to teach.

In illness they struggle on long after many would have given up their duties.

## VINE

Very capable people, certain of their own ability, confident of success.

Being so assured, they think that it would be for the benefit of others if they could be persuaded to do things as they themselves do, or as they are certain is right. Even in illness they will direct their attendants.

They may be of great value in emergency.

## BEECH

For those who feel the need to see more good and beauty

in all that surrounds them. And, although much appears to be wrong, to have the ability to see the good growing within. So as to be able to be more tolerant, lenient and understanding of the different way each individual and all things are working to their own final perfection.

## ROCK WATER

Those who are very strict in their way of living; they deny themselves many of the joys and pleasures of life because they consider it might interfere with their work.

They are hard masters to themselves. They wish to be well and strong and active, and will do anything which they believe will keep them so. They hope to be examples which will appeal to others who may then follow their ideas and be better as a result.

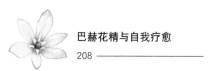

# DIRECTIONS

For those unable to treat themselves or to prepare their own supplies, treatment and remedies can be obtained on application to the Bach Centre.[1]

## METHODS OF DOSAGE[2]

As all these remedies are pure and harmless, there is no fear of giving too much or too often, though only the smallest

---

[1]  With the exception of the longer introduction, dictated by Bach before his death, pages 34 and 35 are the only pages where the 1941 edition differs from the 1936 edition. Nora Weeks edited them to let readers know that remedies (and help choosing them) were also available from the Bach Centre: cf. page 26 of the 1936 facsimile edition at www.bachcentre.com/centre/download/healers1936.pdf.

[2]  The dosage instructions in later editions of *The Twelve Healers* were substantially rewritten to address questions and concerns raised by remedy users. Compare for example pages 23 and 24 of www.bachcentre.com/centre/download/healers.pdf, the Bach Centre's 2009 edition.

quantities are necessary to act as a dose. Nor can any remedy do harm should it prove not to be the one actually needed for the case.

To prepare, take about two drops from the stock bottle into a small bottle nearly filled with water; if this is required to keep for some time a little brandy may be added as a preservative.

This bottle is used for giving doses, and but a few drops of this, taken in a little water, milk, or any way convenient, is all that is necessary.

In urgent cases the doses may be given every few minutes, until there is improvement; in severe cases about half-hourly; and in long-standing cases every two or three hours, or more often or less as the patient feels the need.

In those unconscious, moisten the lips frequently.

Whenever there is pain, stiffness, inflammation, or any local trouble, in addition a lotion should be applied. Take a few drops from the medicine bottle in a bowl of water and in this soak a piece of cloth and cover the affected part; this can be kept moist from time to time, as necessary.

Sponging or bathing in water with a few drops of the

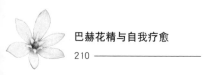
remedies added may at times be useful.

## METHOD OF PREPARATION[①]

Two methods are used to prepare these remedies.

### SUNSHINE METHOD

A thin glass bowl is taken and almost filled with the purest water obtainable, if possible from a spring nearby.

The blooms of the plant are picked and immediately floated on the surface of the water, so as to cover it, and then left in the bright sunshine for three or four hours, or less time if the blooms begin to show signs of fading. The blossoms are then carefully lifted out and the water poured into bottles so as to half fill them. The bottles are then filled up with brandy to preserve the

---

① Towards the end of the 1970s Nora Weeks decided to withdraw a book on remedy-making she had written with Victor Bullen, amid concerns that essences prepared using Bach's methods might be seen as part of his system, regardless of the plants used. Most of this section was removed at the same time. The Bach Centre republished the Weeks & Bullen book in 1998: see the Preface to *The Bach Flower Remedies: Illustrations and Preparations*.

remedy. These bottles are stock[1] , and are not used direct for giving doses. A few drops are taken from these to another bottle, from which the patient is treated, so that the stocks[2] contain a large supply. The supplies from the chemists should be used in the same way.[3]

The following remedies were prepared as above:

Agrimony, Centaury, Cerato, Chicory, Clematis, Gentian, Gorse, Heather, Impatiens, Mimulus, Oak, Olive, Rock Rose, Rock Water, Scleranthus, the Wild Oat, Vervain, Vine, Water Violet, White Chestnut Blossom.[4]

———————————

[1]　Bach refers to mother tinctures as "stock remedies", and makes a dosage remedy directly from the mother tincture. In fact, the normal dilution process involves three stages: energised water mixed with brandy to make mother tincture; mother tincture diluted at the ratio of two drops to 30mls (1 oz.) of brandy to make a stock remedy; and the stock remedy then diluted before taking as described in the section on Dosage. It isn't clear why Bach only refers to two stages in this passage, but it's likely that he didn't consider the middle stage necessary for people who were making small quantities for personal use.

[2]　For "stocks" read "mother tinctures" – see previous note.

[3]　The supplies from the chemists would have been standard-strength stock remedies.

[4]　"White Chestnut Blossom" is so called to differentiate it from the buds of the same tree, used to prepare Chestnut Bud. See The Boiling Method below.

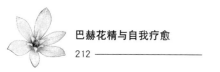
Rock Water. It has long been known that certain wells and spring waters have had the power to heal some people, and such wells or springs have become renowned for this property. Any well or any spring which has been known to have had healing power and which is still left free in its natural state, unhampered by the shrines of man, may be used.

## THE BOILING METHOD

The remaining remedies were prepared by boiling as follows:

The specimens, as about to be described, were boiled for half an hour in clean pure water.

The fluid strained off, poured into bottles until half filled, and then, when cold, brandy added as before to fill up and preserve.

Chestnut Bud. For this remedy[1] the buds are gathered from the White Chestnut tree, just before bursting into leaf.

In others the blossom should be used together with small pieces of stem or stalk and, when present, young fresh leaves.

---

[1] The 1941 edition has "remdy"; we have corrected to "remedy", which is what was in the 1936 edition.

All the remedies given can be found growing naturally in the British Isles, except Vine, Olive, Cerato, although some are true natives of other countries along middle and southern Europe to northern India and Tibet.

The English and botanical name of each remedy is as follows:

| | | |
|---|---|---|
| * AGRIMONY | . | *Agrimonia Eupatoria* [1] |
| ASPEN . | . | *Populus Tremula* |
| BEECH . | . | *Fagus Sylvatica* |
| * CENTAURY | . | *Erythræa Centaurium* [2] |
| * CERATO | . | *Ceratostigma Willmottiana* [3] |

---

[1]　The convention with the Latin names of plants is to capitalise the first word and not the second:*Agrimonia eupatoria*. In early editions of *The Twelve Healers and Other Remedies* both parts of the Latin names were capitalised, and we have left this uncorrected.

[2]　The Latin name given to a plant is governed by the International Code for Botanical Nomenclature. The rules used change from time to time, and some of the names in the 1941 text are now out of date. The modern name of the plant used to make the Centaury remedy, for example, is *Centaurium umbellatum*.

[3]　The Greek word-ending-*ma* is not in fact feminine, and the correct Latin name for this plant is *Ceratostigma willmottianum*. We have retained *willmottiana* here as it is so widely used in books on the remedies.

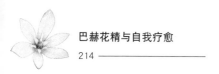

| CHERRY PLUM | . | *Prunus Cerisfera* |
| CHESTNUT BUD | . | *Æsculus Hippocastanum* |
| * CHICORY | . | *Cichorium Intybus* |
| * CLEMATIS | . | *Clematis Vitalba* |
| CRAB APPLE | . | *Pyrus Malus* [1] |
| ELM . | . | *Ulmus Campestris* [2] |
| * GENTIAN | . | *Gentiana Amarella* |
| GORSE . | . | *Ulex Europæus* |
| HEATHER | . | *Calluna Vulgaris* |
| HOLLY . | . | *Ilex Aquifolium* |
| HONEYSUCKLE | . | *Lonicera Caprifolium* |
| HORNBEAM | . | *Carpinus Betulus* |
| * IMPATIENS | . | *Impatiens Royleii* [3] |
| LARCH . | . | *Larix Europea* [4] |
| * MIMULUS | . | *Mimulus Luteus* [5] |
| MUSTARD | . | *Sinapis Arvensis* |

[1] The modern name is *Malus pumila* .
[2] Modern name *Ulmus procera.*
[3] Modern name *Impatiens glandulifera* .
[4] Modern name *Larix decidua.*
[5] Modern name *Mimulus guttatus* .

| | | |
|---|---|---|
| OAK . | . | *Quercus Pedunculata* [1] |
| OLIVE . | . | *Olea Europæa* |
| PINE . | . | *Pinus Sylvestris* |
| RED CHESTNUT | . | *Æsculus Carnea* |
| * ROCK ROSE | . | *Helianthemum Vulgare* [2] |
| ROCK WATER . | | |
| * SCLERANTHUS | . | *Scleranthus Annuus* |
| STAR OF BETHLEHEM | | *Ornithogalum Umbellatum* |
| SWEET CHESTNUT . | | *Castanea Vulgaris* [3] |
| * VERVAIN . | | *Verbena Officinalis* |
| VINE . | . | *Vitis Vinifera* |
| WALNUT | . | *Juglans Regia* |
| * WATER VIOLET . | | *Hottonia Palustris* |
| WHITE CHESTNUT | | *Æsculus Hippocastanum* |
| WILD OAT . | | *Bromus Asper* †[4] |
| WILD ROSE . | | *Rosa Canina* |
| WILLOW . | | *Salix Vitellina* |

——————————

[1]  Modern name *Quercus robur* .

[2]  Modern name *Helianthemum nummularium* .

[3]  Modern name *Castanea sativa* .

[4]  Modern name *Bromus ramosus* .

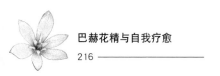
† There is no English name for Bromus Asper.[1] Bromus is an ancient word meaning Oat.

---

① This footnote on Wild Oat is part of the 1941 text.

And may we ever have joy and gratitude in our hearts that the Great Creator of all things, in His Love for us, has placed the herbs in the fields for our healing.

巴赫花精植物彩图

由英国巴赫中心提供

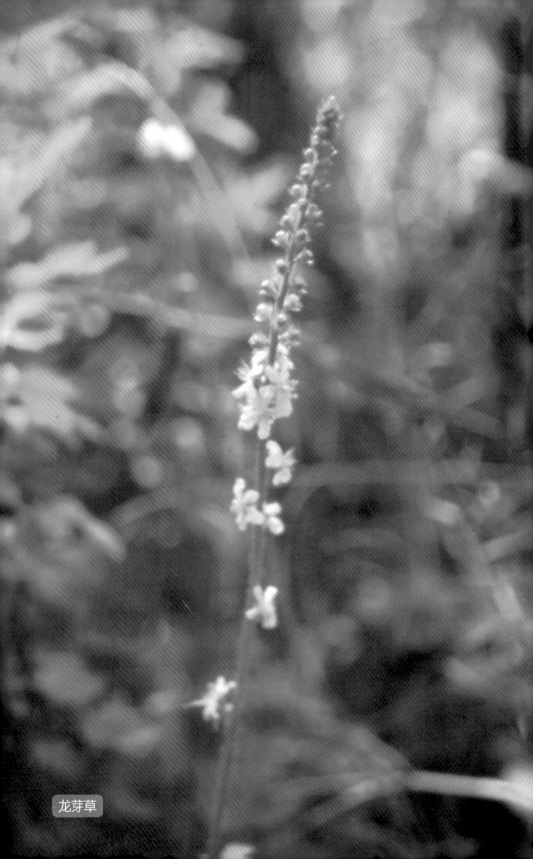

龙芽草

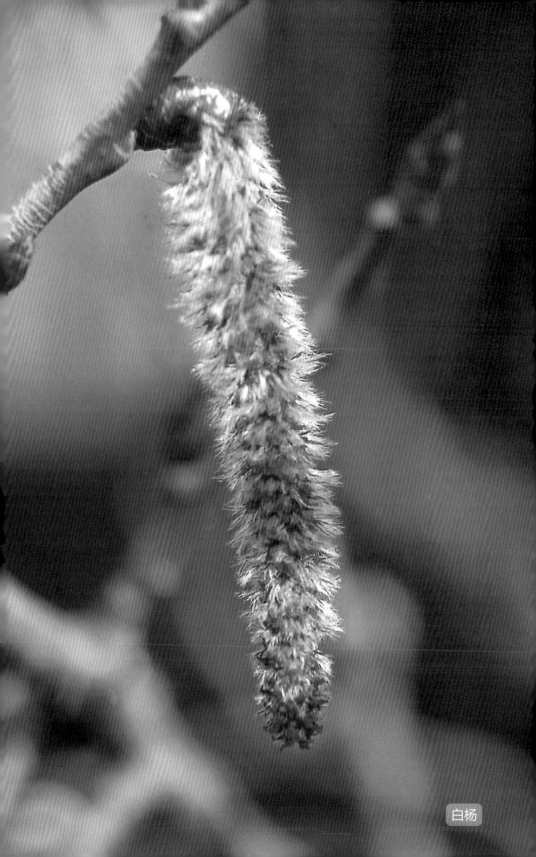
白杨

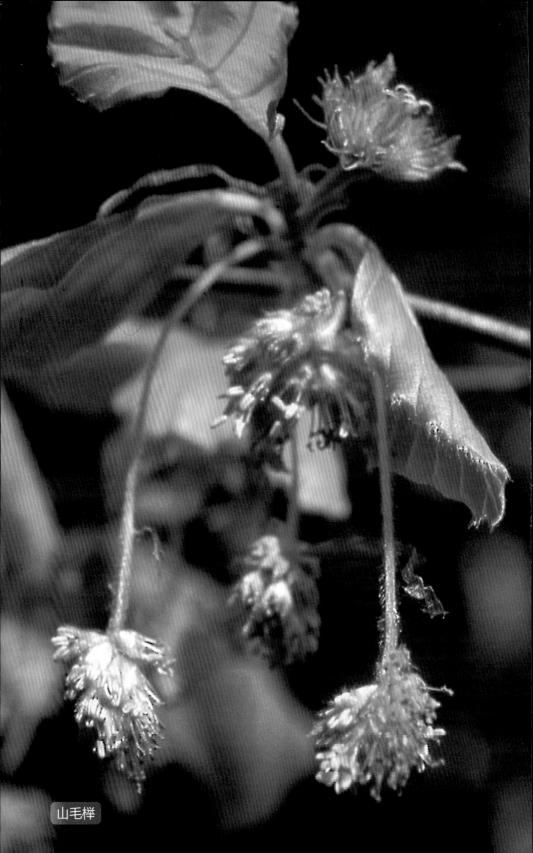
山毛榉

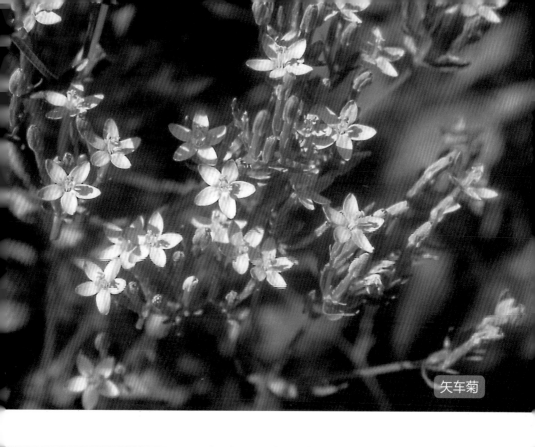
矢车菊

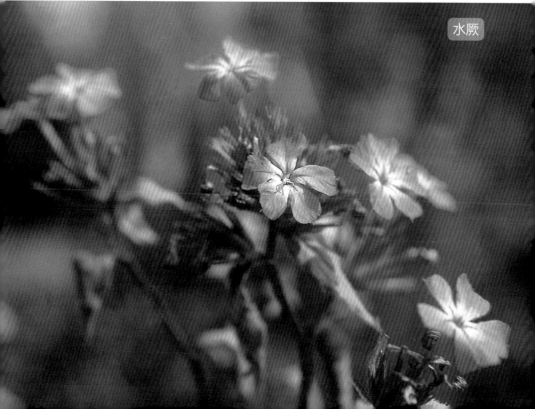
水厥

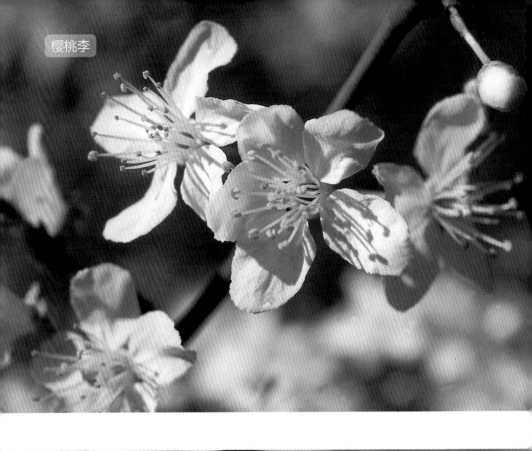

櫻桃李

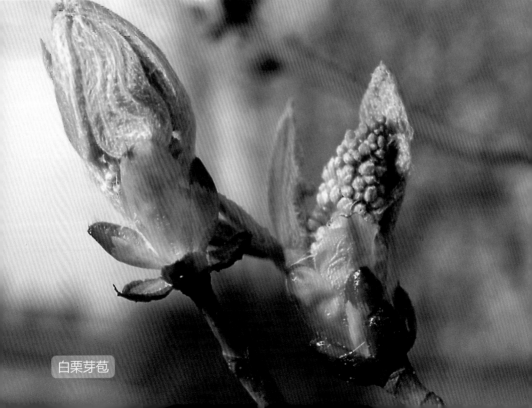

白栗芽苞

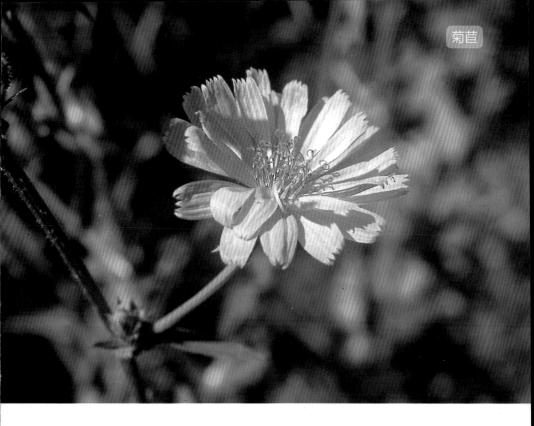
菊苣

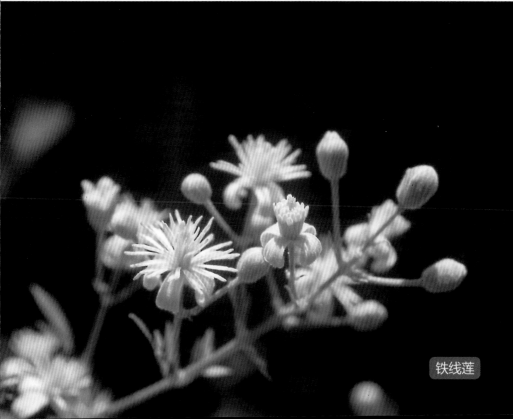
铁线莲

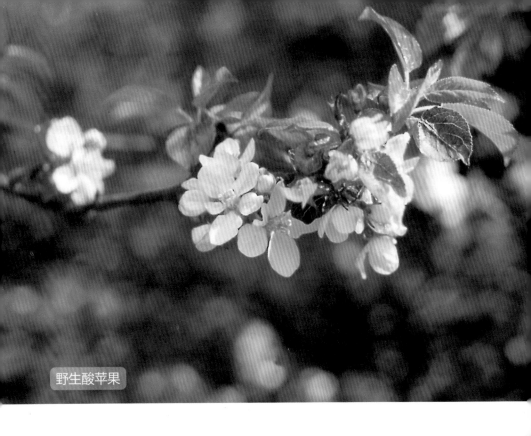

野生酸苹果

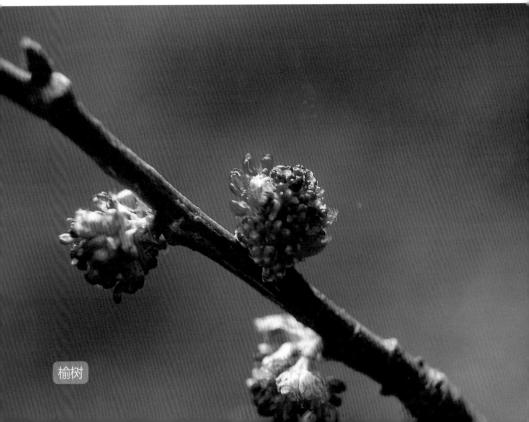

榆树

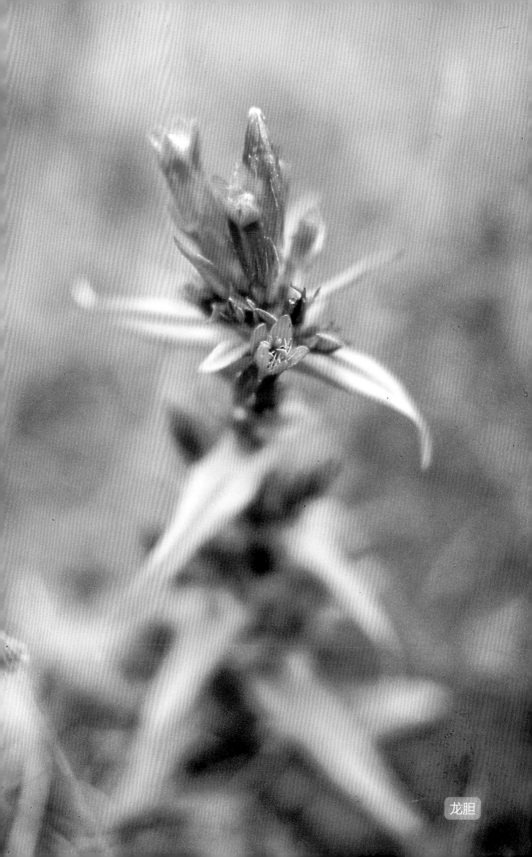
龙胆

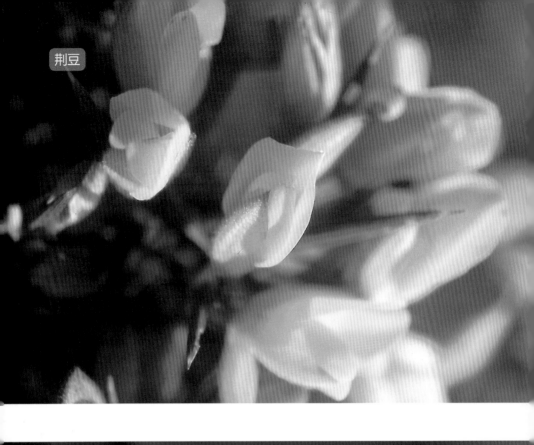

荆豆

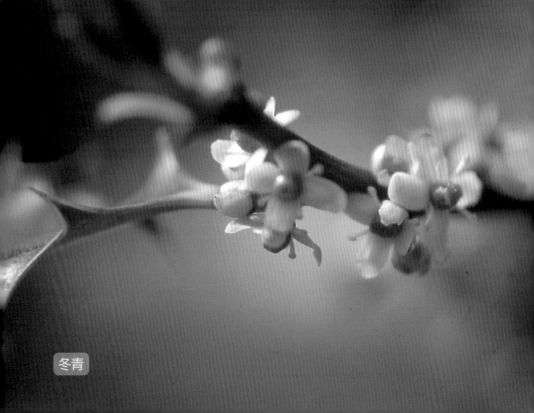

冬青

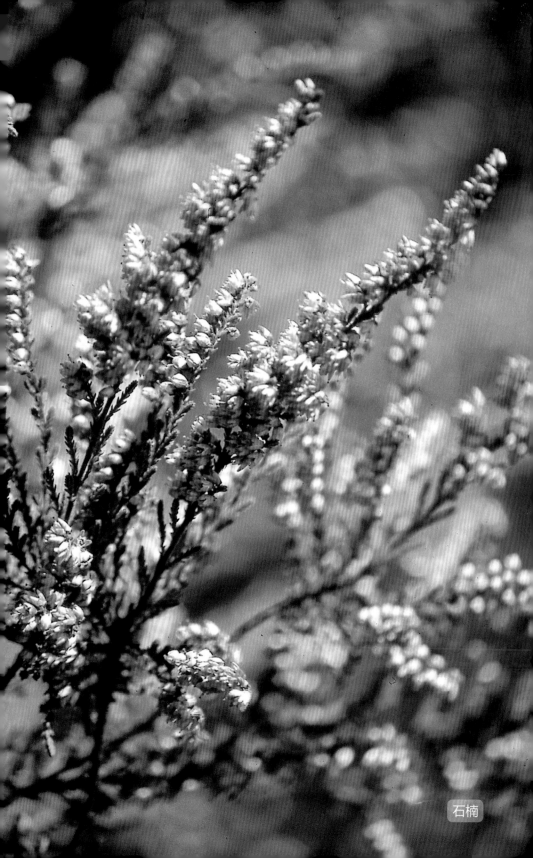
石楠

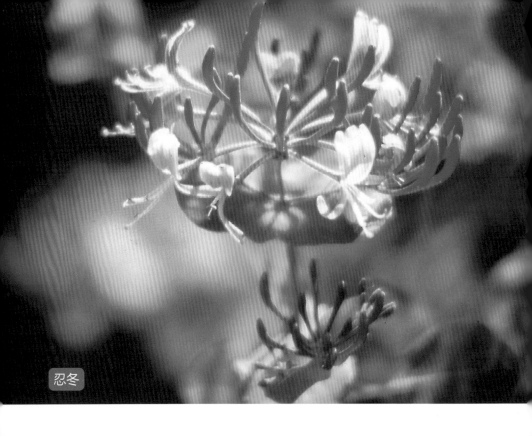

忍冬

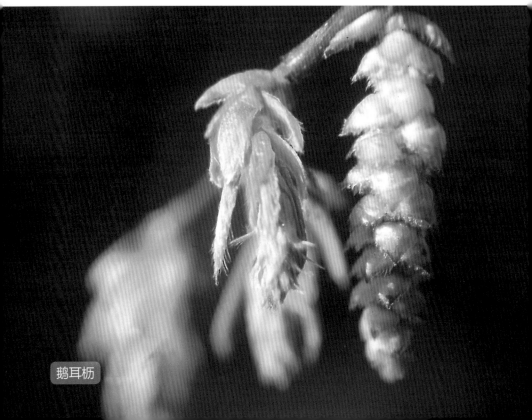

鹅耳枥

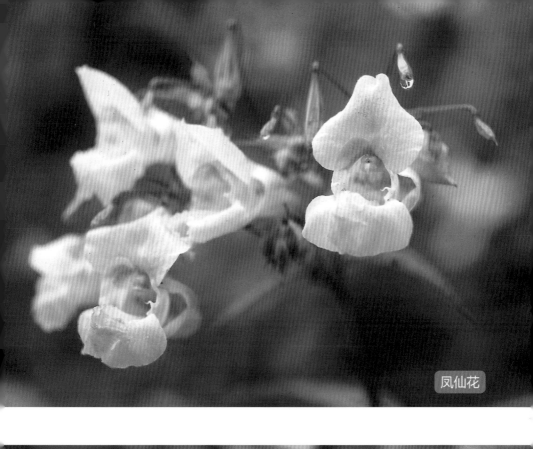

凤仙花

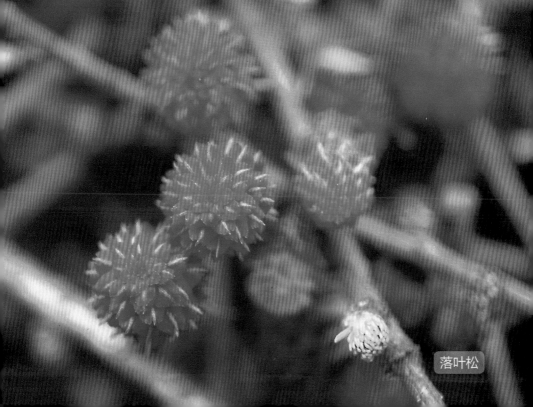

落叶松

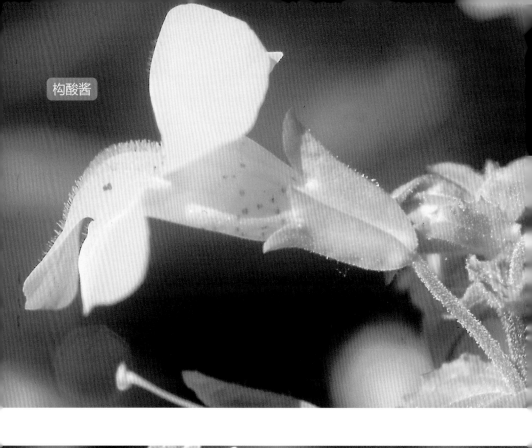

构酸酱

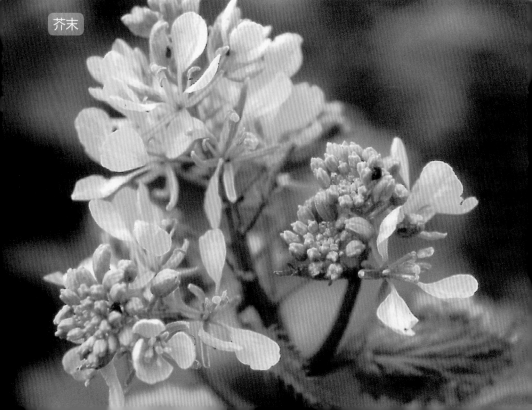

芥末

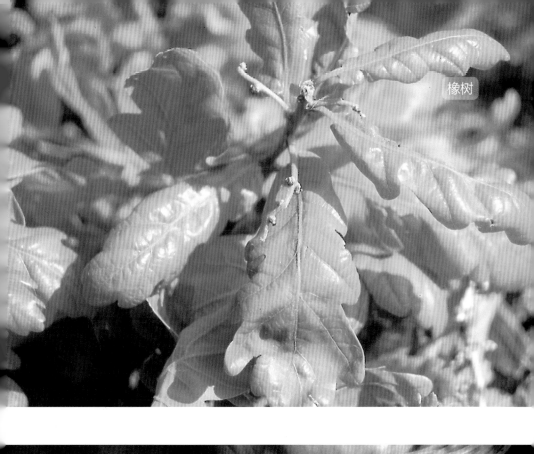

橡树

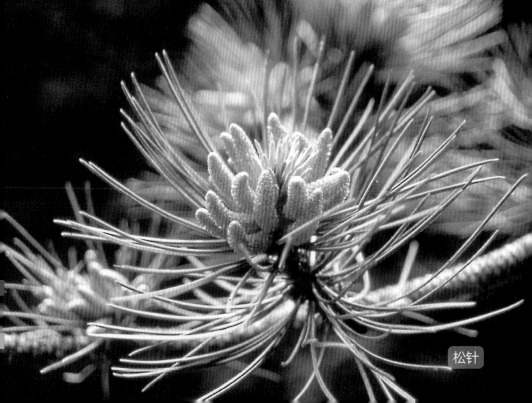

松针

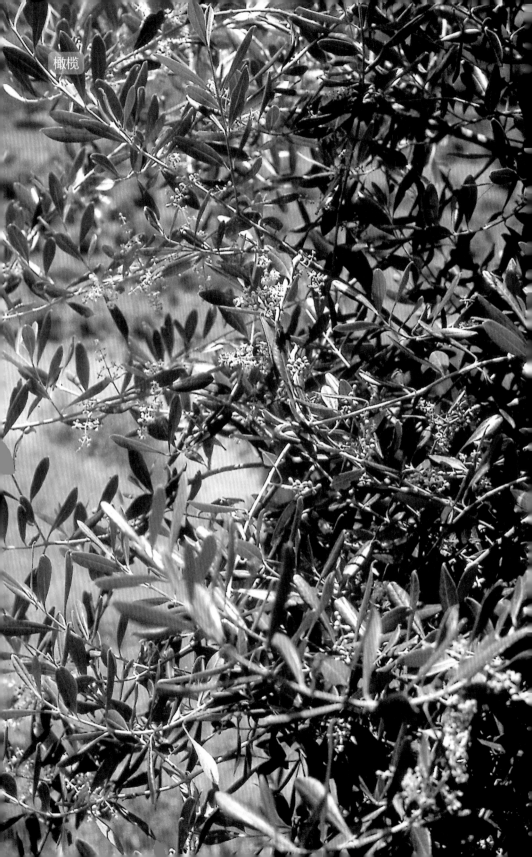

橄榄

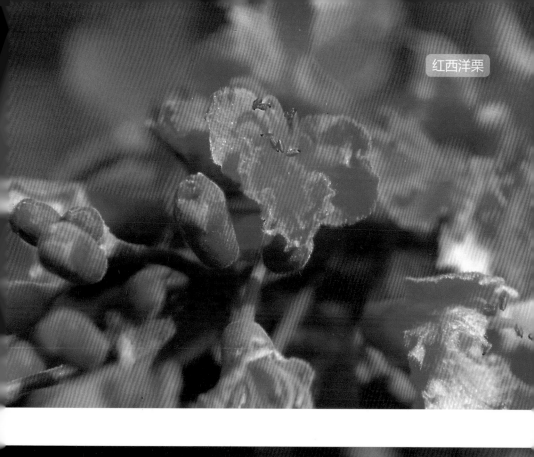

红西洋栗

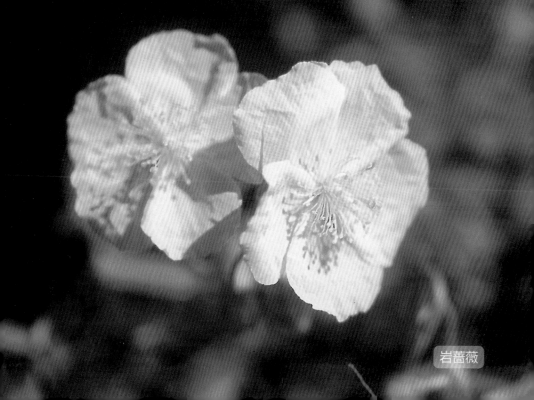

岩蔷薇

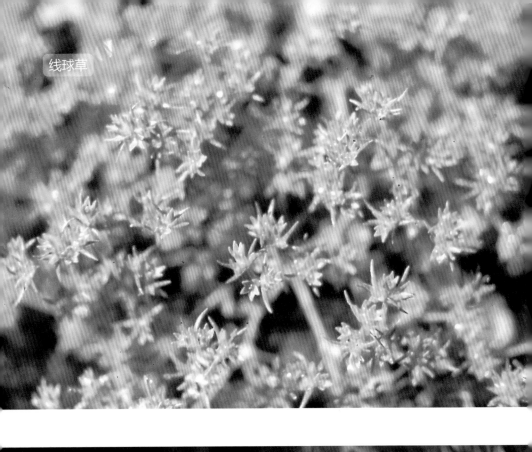

线球草

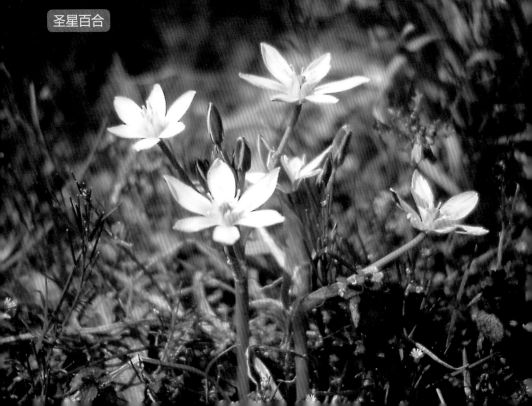

圣星百合

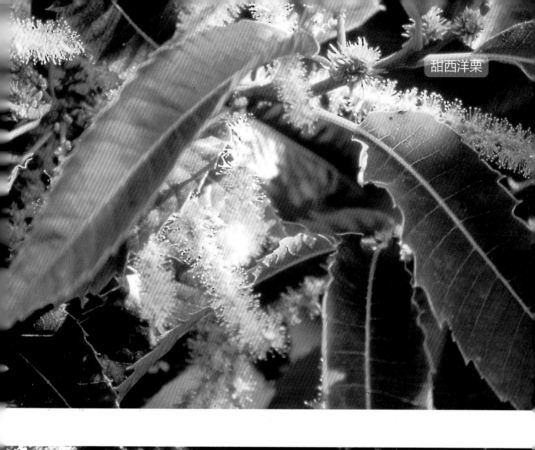

甜西洋栗

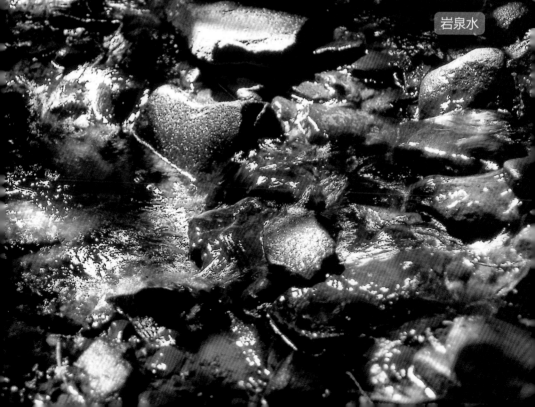

岩泉水

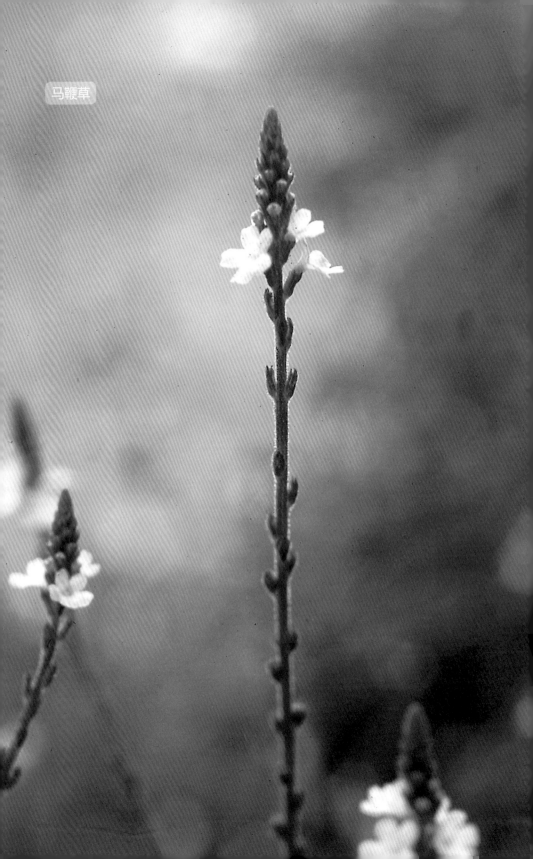

马鞭草

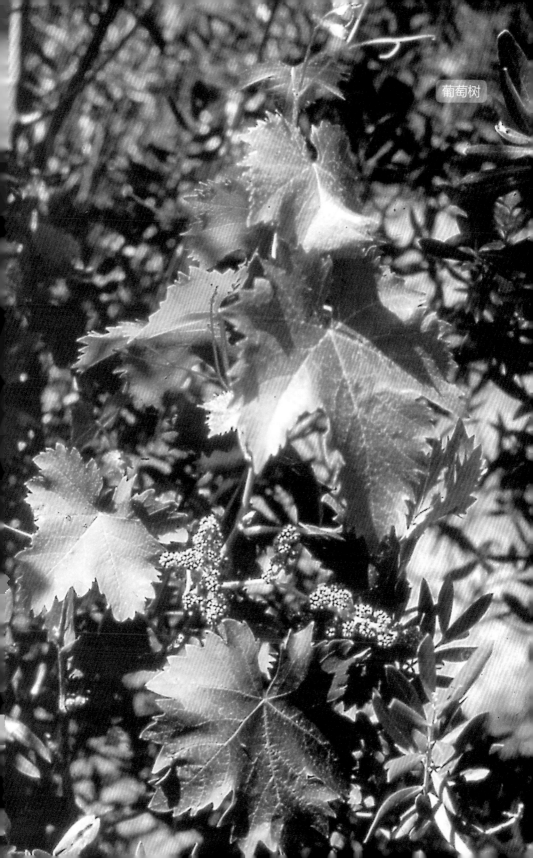

葡萄树

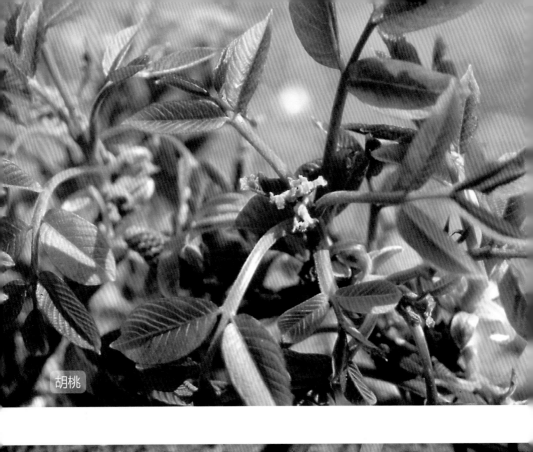

胡桃

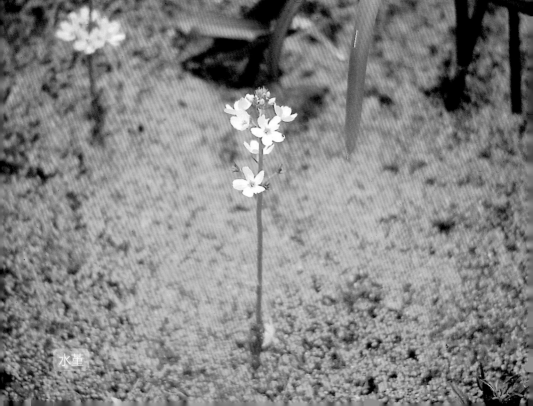

水堇

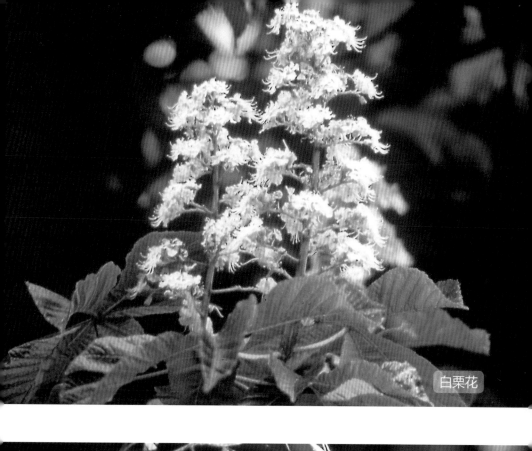

白栗花

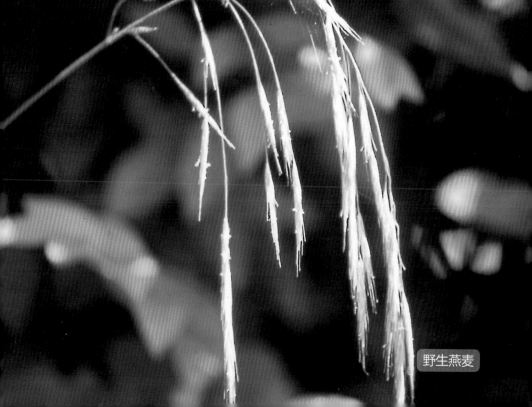

野生燕麦

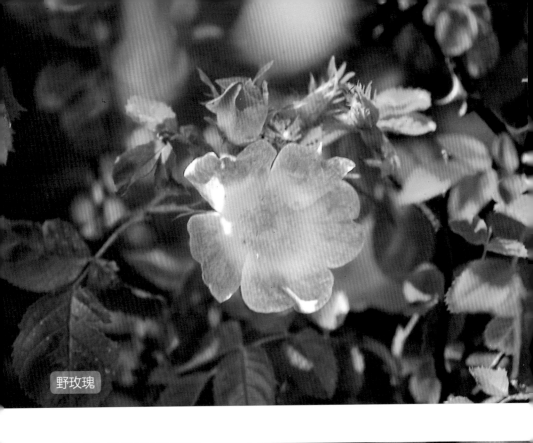

野玫瑰

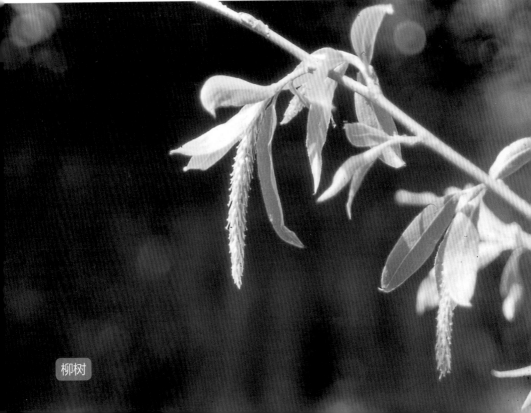

柳树